#5
10/24

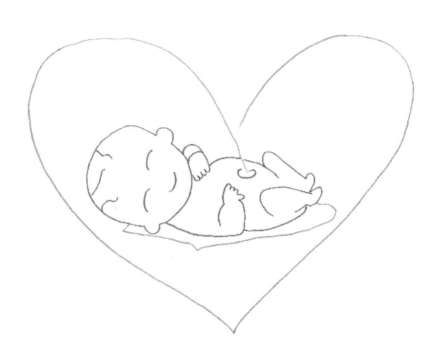

GARBH SANSKAR

*Ancient secrets to give
birth to genius*

JUHI SOHAL

First Edition
April, 2022
Printed in India
Edited by Ashish Kollamparambil
ashiskb@gmail.com

Published by Juhi Sohal
Officialsupermoms@gmail.com

Interior Illustrations © 123rf (Page 7), Vectorstock (Pages 19, 35, 134, 142, 155, 176), Vectorportal (Page 54), WDRfree (Page 88), Google Images (Pages 20, 100, 113, 115, 116, 128, 170), Shutterstock (Pages 113, 114, 116, 149, 157), Adobestock (Page 151), Freepik (Page 140), Pixlr (Page 151), Dreamstime (Page 151), Seekpng (Page 151) and Insightsdice (Page 151).

FOR
ALL THE MOMS WHO HAVE RESOLVED TO
GIVE THEIR BEST TO THEIR BABIES AND
MAKE THIS WORLD A BETTER PLACE

I WANT TO DEDICATE THIS BOOK TO MY
MOTHER WITH DEEP RESPECT AND LOVE.
YOU NOT ONLY GAVE ME THE GIFT OF
LIFE BUT AN UNRELENTING PASSION FOR
BECOMING MY BEST VERSION AND
SERVING SOCIETY. I AM VERY GRATEFUL
TO YOU.

PREFACE

A mother is a portal through which new life comes on this planet. While giving birth is no less than a miracle, the process can sometimes feel challenging and overwhelming. In the flow of life, it might feel like a natural routine event. Motherhood can be extraordinary and ordinary simultaneously.

When a woman learns about her pregnancy, the thoughts of baby's health, well-being and overall development occupy her mind.

Every mother wants the best for her baby. I was one such mother.

My curiosity took me to the history of Ancient India and I came across the practice of 'Garbh Sanskar.' Garbh Sanskar finds its mention in the Vedas and Upanishads as well. After extensive research, I realized that the baby's life depends substantially on how a pregnant woman spends her pregnancy.

In the past, women were aware of this ancient technique of Garbh Sanskar and practiced it diligently. This resulted in the birth of strong, healthy and happy babies. However, this practice has been lost with time, like many other practices.

When a woman is pregnant, she has the power equivalent to the mother nature. She can inculcate all the virtues in the baby right from her womb. When a mother takes care of these nine months consciously, she can give birth to a baby with a higher Intelligence Quotient(IQ), Emotional Quotient (EQ), Spiritual Quotient (SQ), and Adversity Quotient (AQ).

Through this book, I want to create awareness about Garbh Sanskar amongst planning and expecting couples for their baby's best development. When a mother becomes aware, she can create a masterpiece. Let's make this world a better place together.

AUTHOR'S NOTE

Through this book, I want to help you make your pregnancy journey happy, healthy, peaceful and full of positivity. You will learn certain rituals which, on consistent practice, will help you instill virtues in your baby right from the womb and give birth to a genius - his best version physically, mentally, emotionally and spiritually. You will develop a deeper bond with your baby even before he is born.

Please note: For a better understanding of readers, I have chosen to explain the 'Garbh Sanskar' in the form of a story. Further, for a quick reference, the page numbers of the crucial non-fictional elements are mentioned as subpoints under the contents section of the book.

The characters – Ananya, Riya, Ancient Guru and others, are all fictional characters and are a result of my imagination. However, 'Garbh Sanskar' is a real practice that wise women have practiced for 5000 years. It will help you attract all the qualities you desire in your baby. Legends were born on this planet through this ancient secret of Garbh Sanskar.

For the ease of reading, I have addressed the baby as 'he' in the book. You can address the baby as 'she' if it connects with you. Further, certain rituals include lighting a lamp, chanting OM, reciting Sanskrit shlokas, etc. They are included for the proven benefits they possess and are by no means meant to promote or offend any particular religion. Feel free to modify the rituals as per your beliefs and customs.

The term 'Divine' has been often mentioned in the book. All I am trying to convey through the word Divine is the existence of certain energies that are our allies and work for our growth. If it makes you uncomfortable, you can call it angels, muse, god, or higher power. You can even think of them as something impersonal like the law of gravity.

The journey of motherhood starts from the very first thought of having a baby. It would be of tremendous help if a woman starts making lifestyle changes immediately after she thinks about conceiving a baby. The scope of this book is limited to the things which a woman must do in her pregnancy but she can start practicing these rituals in the pre-pregnancy phase too.

For all the husbands feeling FOMO, your presence in her pregnancy journey plays a crucial role in your baby's best development. You can support your wife in practising her rituals. You can accompany her for walks, create music playlists, read books with her, play with her, solve puzzles with her, be creative, start gardening, work out and meditate with her; cook for her and with her; and make her feel loved and valued. Talk with your baby in the womb to nurture a deeper bond. Pamper her and take good care of her. Give her your best so that she can be her best version and give birth to a genius baby.

"No language can express the power and beauty and heroism of a mother's love." — **Edwin Chapin.**

"One good mother is worth a hundred schoolmasters." — **George Herbert.**

"Birth is the epi-centre of women's power." — **Ani DiFranco.**

"Babies are bits of star-dust blown from the hand of God. Lucky the woman who knows the pangs of birth for she has held a star." — **Larry Barretto.**

CONTENTS

ACKNOWLEDGMENTS

I am very fortunate to have tremendous blessings in my life, one of them being my Gurudev Sri Sri Ravi Shankar. I am very grateful to many people in the making of this book. But, first, I would like to express my gratefulness to the magical world of Art of Living which I am blessed to be a part of.

I am thankful to my mom, who has always stood by my side. She has always been my pillar of strength.

To Vipin for supporting my author's journey.

To Jaival for being so adorable and taking my stress away with that beautiful smile.

To Sweta Samota for making book writing possible.

To Ashish Kollamparambil for editing my book and spending several hours on discussions.

To Anant Agrawal for reviewing my first draft and giving valuable suggestions.

To Dr. Chandrakant Amdavadi for introducing me to the ancient secrets of Garbh Sanskar and ayurvedic dincharya.

To Dr. Shivani Billimoria for always inspiring me to be my best version.

To Dr. Prashul for listening to my thoughts on the book.

To Dr. Hemant Sharma for introducing me to Marma Therapy.

To Dr. Deepa Kaushik for showing the power of Garbh Samvad.

To Dr. Shital Lathiya for always showing me the right path in Garbh Sanskar.

To Vrunda Maa for teaching the science of mudras.

To Asheeh Pal for the excellent analogy on types of bodies.

To Nilima Kanth for the knowledge of microgreens.

To Geetika Saigal for the book writing techniques.

To Sejal Thakkar for Agnihotra Homa.

To Meghavi Desai for teaching me transcendental meditation.

To Tushita Rathod for showing me the power of positive affirmations.

To Kamlesh Barwal for always uplifting my energy.

To Shivam for encouraging me to write this book.

To Twinkle Desai for always encouraging me in all my endeavours.

And to you, dear readers, thank you for buying this book and reading it. Enjoy your Garbh Sanskar journey!

Sending lots of positive energy,
All the Best,
Juhi Sohal

PROLOGUE

There were two stripes on the 'prega test' kit. Ananya couldn't believe her eyes. It felt surreal. She was ecstatic and anxious at the same time. Her happiness knew no bounds. She couldn't believe that it was finally happening. Every cell of her body was dancing with happiness. She went to Arjun and put his hand on her belly, nodding in affirmation. Arjun was delighted to learn that their wait was finally over and his wife Ananya was now pregnant again. After her first miscarriage five years back, they had been longing to see this. Arjun and Ananya had all the worldly things that money could buy but deep down, they had been feeling empty. They were feeling the void created in their hearts was due to the absence of children in their lives, which they had both desired for years.

After knowing that she was pregnant again, she couldn't help but think of her past. All her childhood memories of conflicts between her parents and finally their separation when she was just eight came before her eyes. As she was a single child, she had a painful and lonely childhood. She always thought that she would have a perfect family, safeguard her baby from everything she had gone through, and do whatever it takes for her baby's best development and happiness. So, the same day, she started her extensive research on what a pregnant woman should do for the baby's best growth. She also booked an appointment with her gynecologist, Dr. Rita, to confirm the pregnancy. Being a lawyer, she wanted to be sure as she had to have a proof for everything. Her analytical mind didn't let her rest completely. She was very sensitive and would stress out very quickly.

Ananya spent most of her time in her office, helping her clients win their cases. She worked in LawFirst – one of the top law firms in India. She also participated in free legal aid camps to help people in distress. She disliked wearing traditional dresses and skirts and always wore a white shirt and formal black pants at work. Last week, she had won a case of one of her clients in which the defendant had forged her clients' trademark. She proved before the jury that the trademark originally belonged to her client, and judgment was given in her client's favor after heated arguments. When justice was served, it gave her deep satisfaction and this was her way of serving society.

Later, Ananya grabbed a burger and car keys and drove to Dr. Rita's clinic to confirm her pregnancy. She frequently used to eat while traveling to save time to do things that mattered the most.

Ananya parked her car and entered the Mamma & Baby Hospital. After talking with the receptionist, Ananya sat cross-legged in Dr. Rita's cabin. She was playing with her long curly hair and tapping her foot on the floor. She wasn't her usual self because today was different. She wanted the results to be positive so badly that she couldn't help but forget to keep her poise and composure as one of the finest corporate lawyers. Dr. Rita looked at the previous records and asked Ananya to lie on the bed and pull her shirt up towards the chest to scan the abdomen for sonography. She clenched her teeth tightly and tensed both her fists while grabbing her shirt. Her breath almost stopped.

"Can you see this tiny black dot on the screen?" asked Dr. Rita.

Ananya nodded.

Dr. Rita turned off the machine and asked her to have a seat. Ananya was sweating profusely and had tiny stress lines on her face. *Is everything alright?* Her heart pounded a thousand times every minute and it felt as if it would explode.

Dr. Rita sensed her anxiety and said, "Ananya, you can relax now. You are four weeks pregnant!"

Ananya finally released her fingers which were tightly holding her handbag.

"Are you sure, doctor?" asked Ananya. *I want to be double sure because this news is no less than a miracle.*

"Yes, Ananya! Congratulations on your new journey," replied Dr. Rita.

Ananya's happiness knew no bounds. All stress lines on her forehead were replaced with a distinct dimple on her right cheek as she smiled through her eyes. In split seconds, the tension in her body turned into enthusiasm.

She asked, "Dr. Rita, can you please suggest what I should be doing for the best development of the baby?"

Dr. Rita said, "You should be happy, eat healthy and nutritious food, take your supplements on time..."

"Please, doctor, these are generic pieces of advice. I know you have been into spirituality for a long time," Ananya declared. "I want him to be joyous, healthy, intelligent, just, curious, fun-loving, etc. What would you recommend me to do for my baby during pregnancy for his best development?"

Dr. Rita looked straight into her eyes to check if she was serious enough. She thought for a moment and said, "Do you want to attract a baby full of virtues, the genius mindset with the best of physical, mental, emotional, and spiritual development?"

"Yes," asserted Ananya.

"It will not be easy but if you are willing to make certain lifestyle changes, then I have something for you," smiled Dr. Rita.

"Yes, I am ready for the change, doctor," declared Ananya.

Dr. Rita looked at Ananya from top to bottom and saw a determined mother. She took her cell phone and called someone. After talking for a while, Dr. Rita returned to Ananya. She told her that she would get to know whatever needs to be done during pregnancy in the mastery sessions. Dr. Rita warned her that it wouldn't be an easy journey, but it will be worth it. She gave a piece of paper to Ananya and bid her goodbye.

Why would it be difficult? Ananya couldn't comprehend. After she sat in her car, she took out that piece of paper. It read, "ANCIENT GURU, Banyan Tree, Greenland Park, Ville at 5 a.m. tomorrow". She had been to the Greenland park before but never this early. It's a beautiful place surrounded by greenery spread across 100 acres with one main Banyan Tree in the center, over 150 years old. It has a small waterfall a few steps ahead of the Banyan tree. The Greenland park was on the city's outskirts, and there was no high-rise building in the vicinity. *Why would someone go there at 5 a.m.?* But she trusted Dr. Rita entirely and was determined to give her baby the best. So, she decided to go there and meet the Ancient Guru.

CHAPTER 1
MEETING THE MASTER

"Everyone can sit on the lush green grass. I know why you all are here. Just settle down and close your eyes", said the Ancient Guru, a man in his 70s who looked no more than 45 years old with a vibrant shine on his face and bald head.

Ananya was mesmerized by the beauty of the place at dawn and regretted why she didn't come here earlier. The park had a few hundred trees. The waterfall was just a few steps away. Its soothing sound was breaking the silence of the dawn. The first rays of the sun were falling on her face, giving it a hue of orange. Beautiful butterflies were flying near the Ancient Guru as if his aura tranquilized them. She saw the Ancient Guru and she suddenly felt a strong gush of positive energy flowing within her. She knew she was at the right place for her pregnancy journey and followed what was instructed.

The Ancient Guru greeted, "Good morning, beautiful ladies! You all are here because you want the best for your baby. All of you wish certain qualities for your baby. These attributes can be broadly classified into four heads:

i.   Happy
ii. Healthy
iii. Successful
iv. Significant

"Do you all agree?" asked the Ancient Guru.

"Yes!" a few women replied from the crowd of more than 3000 women gathered for the session.

"How can you inculcate these attributes in your baby? Do schools and universities guarantee the success of your baby? Or does the gym guarantee perfect health for your baby? Or do religious places guarantee the happiness of your baby?" asked the Ancient Guru and paused for the crowd to answer.

Over 500 women said, "No," and over 300 women answered affirmatively. Others were perplexed.

The Ancient Guru said, "Let's look at it from a different perspective. Today, modern healthcare facilities are improving and becoming more accessible, but our health is deteriorating. Our immunity is weakening. There has been a rise in religious and spiritual places, but our morals are decreasing. Today, we all are connected through social media and the world has become a global village yet people suffer from isolation and depression."

"We all want our children to be successful and significant. Life gets meaning only when it becomes significant. Significance comes by contributing to the betterment of society. Significance comes by improving the lives of other people and doing things for the betterment of the world at large."

The Ancient Guru paused for a while. He stood up from his wooden chair placed on the raised platform under the Banyan tree. His face was radiant in perfect contrast with his maroon kasaya robe and off-white dhoti.

He had a few sips of water from his copper bottle and said, "Today, the world is full of anger, conflicts, violence and arrogance. We will be seeing more of it in the coming years. Would you like to reverse it and give this world peacemakers, humanitarians and great leaders?"

2

A few women said, "Yes."

"Your womb has the power to do this. Today's children are the future of the world. Motherhood is the only portal through which one can enter this world. The most outstanding leaders came to this planet through their mothers' wombs. All the qualities you desire for your baby can be guaranteed by sowing the right seeds. If you want a mango tree, you must sow mango seeds. Expecting the fruits of mango when you sow dates' or apples' seeds is insanity."

A few chuckled. Many were confused.

The Ancient Guru continued,

"You reap what you sow."

"The baby's brain develops very fast in the womb and takes physical, mental, emotional and spiritual clues from his environment through his mother. More than 2,50,000 cells develop in the baby's brain every minute[i]. Due to this rapid division and development of the cells in the fetus, whatever a mother does during her pregnancy, it has the potential to manifest thousand times over."

"When you sow the seeds of happiness, peace, calmness, centeredness, excellence in your womb, it manifests **1000x**. On the other hand, if you sow seeds of anger, frustration, stress, sadness, then all these negative emotions will manifest 1000x in your baby," the Ancient Guru said. "So here we have a chance of a miracle. Either give your all in and contribute towards making this world a better place or relax back and let things take their course. But, do remember improvement can be made in the seeds and not in the trees."

Few ladies in the crowd convulsed. More than 3000 women had gathered in the park to attend the Ancient Guru's session.

Amongst them, half were visibly pregnant, which meant they had less time to implement whatever the Guru guided. Some were just curious to know about the session. However, some women were determined to give the best to their babies.

"Let me tell you something interesting," the Ancient Guru said. "Did you know that it's not you who choose the baby, but it's the baby who chooses you? **The soul chooses the womb conducive to its goal.** The mother with higher prana energy will attract a similar soul with high prana energy and vice versa. The baby you attract depends entirely on you and your current state of mind," the Ancient Guru raised both hands and spread them towards the crowd from inside out.

"Because of lifestyle changes such as disturbed sleep cycle, increased screen time, diet, stressed mind, we all have become weaker in all the aspects of our existence – physical, mental, emotional and spiritual. And the result is that the world we live in today – an aggressive, mentally disturbed, and violent world."

"Pregnancy is the best phase in a woman's life. It is the golden period, an opportunity to contribute to society. The mother attains the position of creator during pregnancy. She has the same power as that of mother nature during this phase[ii]. She can inculcate all the attributes she desires in the baby by just making a few lifestyle changes and following certain rituals consistently during her pregnancy. Mother has the power to attract the best soul and instill attributes of greatness, justice, joyfulness, kindness, humbleness, brilliance, happiness and mindfulness in the baby. If she takes care of nine months of pregnancy, a mother can give birth to a genius baby and make this world a better place to live in."

GENIUS BABY = His Best Version

Physically + Mentally + Emotionally + Spiritually

4

The Ancient Guru scanned the crowd and continued, "Most parents focus on the upbringing of their children after they are born. That is delayed parenting. They chose the best schools and universities for their kids. But sadly, they neglect the most crucial phase in a child's development – 'the pregnancy.' The work done during pregnancy is more potent than any work done for the next 100 years for the baby's development. And most parents, out of lack of awareness or inability to commit to rituals, fail to give their best during that phase."

"Babies take all the clues from the mother while in the womb. Whatever the mother eats, the baby eats through amniotic fluid. Generally, mothers focus just on the baby's physical well-being. Whereas a baby's existence is at all four levels – physical, mental, emotional, and spiritual. The baby is continuously taking mental, emotional, and spiritual clues also. Whenever a pregnant woman gets angry, the baby also learns to get angry in similar situations. He learns whether to react or stay calm, through his mother. When a mother becomes aware, she can send positive energy, thoughts and signals to the baby and give birth to a genius who can impact the world and make it a better place to live."

Someone started whistling and clapping amongst the women gathered at Greenland park. She was full of enthusiasm and vigor. All eyes now turned at her. Riya smiled at everyone with that spark in her eyes. She was a homemaker and a mother of a three-year-old girl. Her wheatish skin and dark brown long straight hairs were complimenting her peach long kurti and white pants. She got to know about her pregnancy a week back and one of her distant relatives told her about the Ancient Guru. Riya was very extroverted and loved to express her emotions. She was all ears when the Ancient Guru was speaking and her mind was absorbing every word he said. It was as if the words were making the cells of her body dance. She could no longer control her excitement and started whistling at the revelation of astounding knowledge.

A few skeptic women made faces. Most of the women didn't mind the gesture.

The positive atmosphere became more positive on the enthusiastic gesture of Riya and the Ancient Guru spoke further, "You all might be wondering how can you sow the better seeds? How can you attract the best soul in the womb?"

"Hmm," a few women responded.

"It is possible through the ancient technique of Garbh Sanskar, which find it's mention in the Vedas and Upanishads. Today even several scientific pieces of research have proven its benefits[iii]. Many women gave birth to the legends through Garbh Sanskar."

"Do you want to know what Garbh Sanskar is?" asked the Ancient Guru.

"Yes," answered the crowd in unison.

"Before that, let's look into what does Sanskar means?" said the Ancient Guru.

"Sanskaras are the values that we want in our children. The list can be different for different people. But, for everyone, they are a positive list of qualities they wish to inculcate in their children, such as happiness, respect for elders, non-violence, calmness, discipline, obedience, etc. Do you all agree?

"Yes!" the crowd shouted.

"Garbh means womb. So, in layman's language,

GARBH SANSKAR MEANS GIVING VIRTUES TO THE BABY IN THE WOMB.[iv]"

"Garbh Sanskar is every emotion you feel, every thought you think, every action you take, every habit you build during your pregnancy."

DID YOU KNOW

? Every minute over 2,50,000 neurons are formed in the fetus's brain to reach 100 billion neurons at the time of delivery.

? The nerve cells in the brain of a baby are equivalent to the total number of stars present in the Milky way galaxy.

? A human brain forms 300 trillion connections to perform all the tasks.

? From 0 – 3 years, the baby brain produces over 1 million new neural connections every second. That's twice

"If a mother is happy throughout her pregnancy, positive and healthy fetus cells are developed. But if the mother is stressed and sad, these cells are weak and unhealthy. That is why it is of tremendous importance that a mother becomes super-conscious right from her pregnancy to give the best to her baby."

"We all know that genes are transferred from the parents to the baby. So, parents are genetic engineers of their babies. But can you manipulate these genes?" asked the Ancient Guru.

The crowd looked perplexed.

"Yes! You can selectively choose the healthy genes in your baby through the science of '*Epigenetics*'.' It is the science that studies how environmental influences lead to the rearrangement of the genes in DNA. This rearrangement of genes due to the experiences of the baby changes the

7

expression of genes, resulting in different behavior in the baby. And you can actually choose this arrangement by changing the experiences of the baby," said the Ancient Guru.

"The laws of evolution always want to activate the positive genes in the baby and suppress the harmful ones. But, for epigenetics to work, you need to make certain changes in your lifestyle. You need to work on your food, thoughts, emotions and habits for nature to work in your favor. Parents are, in reality, 'Genetic Architects.' That is why these nine months of pregnancy are very important. Whatever you do during your pregnancy will manifest 1000x in the baby as more than 2,50,000 cells are developing every minute and genes are being chosen by nature through epigenetics."

The jaws of many women dropped. They looked at each other astounded.

"And you are not the first to try this ancient technique of Garbh Sanskar. As the word suggests, it has been practiced since immemorial times. For thousands of years, wise women have practiced Garbh Sanskar and served society. Garbh Sanskar is like one of those universal laws like the law of gravity. Whether you believe in gravity or not, it will have its effect. Similarly, whether you believe in the Garbh Sanskar or not, it will have its impact. Let's have a glance at the history[vi]:"

1. Abhimanyu

In Mahabharata, Abhimanyu – the son of Arjuna, learned the art of breaking chakravyaha while he was in his mother's womb - Subhadra. He imbibed the knowledge and applied it when required in his adulthood. He couldn't learn how to come out of it because his mother slept while Arjuna was teaching her. Garbh Sanskar has a profound effect on the baby's brain.

2. Chattarapatti Shivaji

Shivaji Maharaja was one of the strongest leaders from western India. He had a vision of a free Hindu nation. His mother, Jijabai, faced atrocities of Mughals while he was in her womb. Mughals had captured their kingdom and killed his father. But Jijabai demonstrated immense strength, and instead of spending her pregnancy crying over what happened, she exhibited bravery and wished for the liberation of their land from Mughals. She instilled courageousness, patriotism, righteousness, justice, and a burning desire to free people from the atrocities of Mughals, in Shivaji. She said his son would bring back the kingdom and defeat the enemies. He learned bravery by hearing the heroic stories right from the womb. And the rest is history.

3. Napolean Bonaparte

Napolean's father was a military general. During war times, his mother stayed on the war field with his father for most of her pregnancy. His mother initially disliked the war environment but soon became habituated to it; and enjoyed the war techniques and atmosphere. As a result, Napoleon learned all the war skills right from his mother's womb and ruled over the world.

4. Prahalada

King Hiranyakashyap's mother, Ditti, didn't believe in Garbh Saskar due to which demon king was born. However, his wife Kayadhu followed Garbh Sanskar under the guidance of Narada and gave birth to Prahalada. He became Lord Vishnu's devotee through the teachings of Narada. Later, Prahalada ended his father's rule, became a great king, and conquered the three worlds.

9

5. King Alarka

Queen Madalsa is one of the finest examples of the potential of a mother through Garbh Sanskar. She was the queen of Kashi and the wife of King Ritadhwaja. She was a very learned and spiritual woman. Even before conception, she declared the baby's qualities, nature, and abilities. Then she used to think about those qualities during her pregnancy and supported it with related activities and food. She told spiritual stories to her baby while in the womb. In this way, Vikranta, Subhahu and Shatrumardana were born. All of them became saints and left the kingdom. The king requested the queen to give birth to a baby who could look over the kingdom of Kashi after the king. So, Queen Madalsa thought about the qualities of the king that a baby should have and combined it with supporting food and activities and gave birth to Alarka, who later looked after the kingdom. King Alarka was well known as a brave emperor. Through Garbh Sanskar, **a mother can do whatever she desires.**

6. Swami Vivekananda

Bhubaneswari Devi was a devotee of Lord Shiva. In Varanasi, it was customary to pray to Lord Shiva during special or unfortunate events. She lived away from Varanasi and was expecting a baby. She requested her aunt to make the offerings to Lord Shiva daily, and she used to spend her days fasting and meditating. Her entire heart and soul were fixed on Lord Shiva. One night she had a dream in which Lord Shiva told her that he would come on this earth as her child. Soon, she delivered a baby boy and named him Narendranath. Later, Narendranath became world-renowned as Swami Vivekananda. He was one of the most significant social reformers and spiritual personalities. He spread Indian spirituality across the world and inspired millions of people.

10

7. Indira Gandhi

Indira Gandhi was the daughter of Jawaharlal Nehra and Kamala Nehru. They were constantly engaged in politics at the time of her birth. She attained mastery in politics right from the womb and took India to new heights in her political career.

"Amazing, right!! These were some of the prominent personalities who were blessed with determined mothers. They made this world a better place. Now onwards when you see any extraordinary person, try to see the creator - his/her mother and you will have all your answers as to how they are the way they are. If you want to see the baby happy for your whole life, then be wise and take care of these nine months. Whatever you do during your pregnancy, it has the potential to manifest in your baby for his whole life and impact next generations," concluded the Ancient Guru.

The crowd was all ears. There was pin-drop silence in the park.

"If you want to give the best to society if you all want to serve the society, nation, and the world then Garbh Sanskar is one of the answers," said the Ancient Guru.

"Garbh Sanskar is very powerful. **Garbh Sanskar is not easy but it's the right thing to do.** Through Garbh Sanskar, you have the power to not only serve your family but the whole world. With the power equivalent to mother nature, it is the highest responsibility of a mother to craft the best art of her life during her pregnancy. This world is full of conflicts, violence, anger, jealousy, and complaints. You can change this world by bringing more change-makers, peacemakers, and happier human beings."

"Lets' look at an analogy. When good food is cooked, who is appreciated?"

11

"The person who cooks," answered a woman in the second row.

"And when bad food is cooked, who is blamed?" asked the Ancient Guru.

"Again, the person who cooked it," answered a woman from the third row wearing square-shaped sunglasses.

"That's correct! When food is cooked well, the person who cooks receives compliments. When food is poorly cooked, the person who cooked it is at fault. Similarly, when there is a bad painting, the artist is at fault; for bad sculpture, the sculptor is at fault, and for bad children, his mother is at fault. But do we ever take the blame? We never blame ourselves. Whenever a child commits a mistake, we blame the child," explained the Ancient Guru.

"Parents scold their children for being hyperactive, poor at memorizing things, their inability to focus, or not being creative. They are unable to see their fault. The tree depends on the seeds sowed. Planting the neem seeds, then expecting mango fruits is futile. Today, a mother spends her pregnancy gossiping, eating junk food, watching T.V., and complaining. But, she expects her baby to be calm, have extraordinary memory power, be ever happy, etc. In this way, she is being unjust to the baby. **Blaming the children breaks their self-esteem and, at later stages, causes depression.** One can reap only what one sows."

"Every mother has two choices:

i.   Accept the way you are. Accept that you cannot get involved in developmental activities. Accept that since you are not doing anything extraordinary, your baby will not have any exceptional qualities.
OR

12

ii. Become an aware mother and do whatever it takes for the baby's best development. Give birth to a baby full of virtues and make this world a better place to live in. Serve the society through your motherhood."

"Garbh Sanskar is not easy but it's the right thing to do. And it all starts by saying 'YES'. If you think you are one of those determined mothers who want the best for their baby and are willing to do whatever it takes, I invite you to this 8-day journey with me. This journey starts tomorrow at 5 a.m. to bring out the best in you and manifest 1000x in your baby. The way you spend your nine months has the power to change the way your baby lives for ninety-nine years on this planet."

"Sangachadwam."

The Ancient Guru joined his hands and said, "It means unity in harmony. Let's unite in our minds and work for the common cause of baby's best development and betterment of the world. You can use this phrase instead of goodbye to remind yourself of your divine purpose and strengthen your commitment."

He blessed everyone and left.

Ananya still couldn't believe what was revealed to her. All this knowledge was alien to her until now. She was trying to comprehend all the words which hit her ears and in the process, she was sitting very still as if she was in deep meditation. Most of the women had already left the Greenland park. Riya was keenly observing Ananya and she came towards her and asked her if everything was fine.

Ananya looked at Riya and said, "Yeah, just processing the knowledge. It's so deep. It's like a whole new world has opened up to me, and I cannot grasp it completely. It feels so surreal. It's magical."

Riya smiled and said, "Don't worry, it will settle down. When you don't know about something, dive into the unknown and feel the change. Trust that the Divine will take care of everything else."

Ananya said, "Thank you so much for caring. See you tomorrow. By the way, what's your name?"

"Riya and yours?" asked Riya.

"Ananya. I am glad to meet you," said Ananya. And they bid each other goodbye.

Riya cares too much. That's her weakness. She wants the best for everyone and in the process, she sometimes goes overboard, which irritates people around her. It hurts her when people close to her don't give their 100% towards their growth as human beings. She is yet to learn how to manage her emotions – a skill that she needs to master.

Riya goes back home and meets her husband, Varun. He was an easy-going person and worked as a banker. He was tall and a little on the healthier side. He believed that workout and self-growth concepts were alien to him. He worked six days a week in the bank, liked to eat, and relaxed on his couch watching Netflix after his work hours. Varun was very joyful about Riya's pregnancy.

Riya loved Varun a lot, but she couldn't accept his laid-back attitude, and that broke her heart. She wanted Varun to utilize his time in productive activities rather than watching T.V. She shared with him about the Ancient Guru and Garbh Sanskar and Varun said she could do whatever she felt best for the baby. Riya felt content after meeting the Ancient Guru. There was a sense of weird calmness in her, which she hadn't experienced before. She was excited to learn more.

14

GARBH SANSKAR: Ancient secrets to give birth to Genius

DO IT RIGHT

1. Motherhood is the only portal through which one can come into this world.
2. More than 2,50,000 cells develop in the baby's brain every minute. When you sow the seeds of happiness, peace, calmness, centeredness and excellence in your womb, it manifests 1000x.
3. The soul chooses the womb conducive to its goal.
4. A woman has the power equivalent to mother nature during pregnancy.
5. If a mother takes care of nine months of pregnancy, a mother can give birth to a genius baby and make this world a better place to live.
6. The baby exists at all four levels – physical, mental, emotional and spiritual and is continuously clues from his mother.
7. Garbh Sanskar means giving virtues to the baby in the womb
8. Garbh Sanskar is every emotion you feel, every thought you think, every action you take and every habit you build during your pregnancy.
9. A mother can selectively choose the healthy genes in her baby through the science of 'Epigenetics.'
10. Parents are, in reality, genetic architects. Whatever a mother does during her pregnancy will manifest 1000x in the baby as more than 2,50,000 cells are developing every minute and genes are being chosen by nature through Epigenetics
11. A few examples of Garbh Sanskar from history are: Abhimanyu, Chattarapatti Shivaji, Napolean Bonaparte, Prahalada, King Alarka, Swami Vivekananda and Indira Gandhi.
12. Through Garbh Sanskar, a mother can do whatever she desires.
13. Garbh Sanskar is not easy but it's the right thing to do.

CHAPTER 2
THE PRAYER

Ananya and Riya greeted each other good morning as they sat on lush green grass. Ananya saw a super-luxury car parked outside the park. She wondered who could be the owner of one of the most expensive cars in the world. The crowd now had about 2000 women out of 3000 women seated in front of the vast more than 100 years old Banyan tree. The Ancient Guru in, his maroon kasaya, was sitting in sukhasana under the Banyan Tree. He was emitting radiance in the pitch-black darkness of the night. The sun was yet to brighten the world. His every cell was emitting prana as if he was one with the cold breeze flowing softly and the dancing leaves of the Banyan Tree along with the chirping of the birds and burbling of the waterfall. There was something with people working towards a higher purpose. The universe was with those who worked for the betterment of society, leaving behind the ego or I-ness.

The Ancient Guru said, "I am happy to see you all today. Remember, you are here for a **purpose**. That purpose is higher than your petty needs. The purpose is to create a revolution. You all are the Change Makers. I welcome you all to this journey of impacting the whole world through your motherhood. From today onwards, you are '**Light Warriors**.' Getting up early and coming here is not easy. It's not easy to do something different when the people you know live their lives differently. It's not easy to choose the path less traveled or forgotten. It's not easy to trust something which you don't understand completely. Garbh Sanskar is not easy. But still, you are here, with the only motive to give the best to your baby. To do whatever it takes to give him the best. Raise your right hand and pat your back for being here. If you feel like you can pat the back of the person sitting to your right and congratulate them for this bravery."

The crowd was filled with surprise. No one expected the session to be interactive and fun. This simple activity uplifted their energy which was earlier hidden behind their sleepy faces and brought smiles to their faces. Everyone patted the back of the person to their right. Their eyes lit up.

"Can anyone tell me why we are meeting at 5 a.m. and not at any other time?" asked the Ancient Guru.

"Because it's convenient for everyone," answered one lady from the fourth row wearing a dark brown hat.

"Because fewer people are there in the park," said another lady from the first row wearing a long white skirt and blue crop top.

The Ancient Guru laughed, "These were very superficial answers. There was a much deeper and more meaningful reason behind it. Most of you don't wake up this early, right?"

The crowd nodded.

"That's why you could not guess the reason. Waking up at this hour has a different impact on us. Our environment is divided into sattva, rajas, and tamas gunnas. One hour and 36 minutes before sunrise is called **Brahma Muhurat**. Brahma means creator, and muhurat means time[vii]. The environment turns sattvic from tamasic at this hour. The universe guides you towards your highest potential and your body can absorb the most in a sattvic environment. Waking up at this hour positively impacts your mind and body. It gives you clarity and vision for life. Whatever you commit during this time is more likely to succeed. Further, each of us emits energy and influences everyone else on this planet. When you wake up

17

early, this influence is less because 90% of the world is sleeping in your impact area. You will be more powerful, and your productivity will increase tremendously when you schedule activities for this hour. Our body also activates Apana vayu during this time which works towards the excretion of waste materials from our systems. Apana vayu doesn't work after sunrise and that is why most people these days are suffering from digestive issues."

It was an AHA moment for the light warriors. Most of them never thought about waking up early. But today was different. They were not just hearing the knowledge; they were living it. They woke up at 4 a.m. with their energies at their peak. They found it hard to believe that they possessed this tremendous amount of energy that they could feel here in the presence of the Master.

"Do you love the reason for coming here at 5 a.m.? Does it inspire you?" asked the Ancient Guru.

The crowd was spellbound. Few women in the third row started clapping and the rest followed. All the women were very grateful.

"Great energy, my strong mothers! Now let's see what makes this universe? Any guesses?" asked the Ancient Guru.

One woman in the first row said, "The universe is made up of matter."

Riya answered, "Love."

Some other answers were Greed, Power, Stars, Air, etc.

The Ancient Guru smiled and declared, "This universe is made up of billions and billions of atoms at the grossest level. But at the subtle level, it's all energy. Even modern science has the string theory, which supports that the universe is made up of energy vibrating at different frequencies.[viii]"

"Everything in this universe, whether living or non-living, has energy in it. There was a Japanese scientist named **Masaru Emoto**. He subjected the water to different emotions[ix] and studied the water crystal structures under the microscope. He was amazed by the results. Can you believe that there were different structures for different emotions?"

The eyes of many women widen. All the boredom evaporated and the crowd was all ears.

"The crystals were in good shape for positive emotions such as love and gratefulness. And the crystals were in bad shape for negative emotions such as hatred and jealousy. But the best crystals were formed from the feeling of **devotion**[x]."

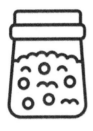

RICE JAR SECRET
Here is a fun experiment for all of you:
Take three glass jars. Fill all of them with 50% rice and 50% with water. Give them tags – Gratitude, Neutral, and Hate. Every day thank the jar tagged as gratitude, stay indifferent with a neutral one, and tell bad words to the hate jar. We will discuss the results on the 7th day.

"Our words, intentions, and thoughts all have energy and are potent weapons that can create or destroy anything. I would like to share with you another example of energy. Africans have an excellent forgiveness ritual[xi]. In Babemba Tribe, if any member acted irresponsibly or unjustly (not the heinous crime like murder, rape, etc.), all the villagers would surround the culprit in a circle and tell all the positive things about that culprit. His positive attributes, good deeds, acts of kindness, and strengths were carefully recited with great detail. After the end of the ceremony, the culprit would be overflowing with emotions of gratefulness. He would regret his wrongdoings and vow never to repeat the mistake. In the end, the celebration would take place and he would be welcomed back into the tribe."

"So, these were some examples of how energy works and why we should be conscious of our thoughts. Our thoughts emit energy. The baby feels this energy. He takes the mental and emotional clues from the mother's thoughts and emotions. And we only want the best to reach the baby in the womb. So, become a super conscious mother this very moment."

"My light warriors, would you like to know our first ritual?" asked the Ancient Guru.

The group of women shouted "yes" in unison.

The Ancient Guru raised his hands and joined them together in front of his chest in namaste mudra. "Our first ritual is 'PRAYER.'"

 RITUAL #1: Pray to Divine Daily

"Now we all know how our emotions affect our baby. We know that everything is energy. Prayer unleashes the highest form of energy[xii]. You will channel positive energy towards your womb and facilitate healthy fetus development by praying daily. Follow this ritual throughout your pregnancy and your baby will be full of devotion. He will be able to quickly surrender the good and the bad and become light from inside. He will have an unshakable faith and centeredness from within."

"Your homework for today is to write a short prayer of 5 – 10 lines in your mother tongue or the language you are most comfortable with and pray to the divine every morning. Surrender your wishes to the divine. You can light an earthen lamp or a candle if your religion permits. Those who are comfortable can also add camphor to their lamp. The camphor vapors are anti-viral, anti-bacterial, and anti-fungal. They have a therapeutic effect on the body and the mind."

"Sangachadwam."

The Ancient Guru blessed everyone and left.

The women were discussing the session and seeing each other's prayer lines. Ananya suddenly realized why Arjun always asked her to focus on positive emotions. It was an AHA moment for her. Now she understood the nature of energy. *Eureka! The energy is contagious.* Whenever someone at work or home didn't do their share of work well, it used to piss her off a lot. So much that she would crib over it a whole day. Arjun always advised that she was wasting her precious day and spoiling the home atmosphere. Still, Ananya would say she was just pointing out the mistakes, and it had nothing to do with the home's ambience. But now she knew how wrong she was. By taking things too seriously and cribbing all the time, she emitted all the negative energy to the atmosphere around her. That influenced Arjun's mood and the people connected with her at home and work.

Today's session reminded her of the day when Arjun proposed to her six years back at the Manera point with the diamond ring. Arjun was a handsome man and owned a payment gateway company DiGi World with a turnover of five crores that year. Ananya was very happy. That day, she vividly remembered being so energetic and enthusiastic despite being stuck in traffic for four long hours after work.

The next day, one of her friends was going to meet her at lunch, but she canceled the plan at the last moment. But as

Ananya was delighted due to last night's event and was living in the present moment, the meet cancellation didn't affect her that day which would otherwise hurt her and she would complain about it the whole day.

She heard the voices of women talking about breath-taking sunrise breaking her train of thought. She now knew that everything was energy, and it was in her hands whether to focus on the positive or the negative energy. She joined the other women and saw the mesmerizing sunrise, taking a fresh breath of positivity.

SAMPLE PRAYERS

Prayer is the most powerful state of energy. Words of prayer can fill you with immense energy. Words of prayer can take you closer to the divine. Through prayer, you can send your message to the divine. When you pray for your baby, his picture is imprinted on your heart. When you pray, divine energy starts flowing through you. Like nuclear energy is generated through atoms, spiritual energy is generated through prayer. With consistency, a desire for a virtuous child becomes a reality.

Prayer connects you with the most incredible energies of this universe. It connects you to the creator of this universe, strengthens your trust in the divine, and gives more clarity on the qualities of the baby you desire. Praying takes your life to a new dimension. It fills you with gratitude. Let every mother get the gift of the best baby.

1.   **Prayer 1 – Pre-conception**

O Lord
This world is an extension of your dimension
Through me, spread your divinity on this planet
And send your divine fragment on this planet through me

I am eagerly waiting for your divine fragment to come and
grow within me
With all your beauty, your divinity, your potential, your
capabilities, your powers, and your purity
Let me experience you through new life within me

2. Prayer 2 – Pre-conception

O Lord,
I desire to see your shapeless form as new life within me
Through me, let a part of your divinity come on this planet
Through his birth, allow me to serve your divinity
Through your divine touch, allow me to become humble
Allow me to see your purity and divinity through new life
growing within me
Through him, bless me to feel your continuously flowing
divinity
Please accept my prayer

3. Prayer 3 – Post-conception

O Lord,
I can feel your blessing growing within me
I can see you showering your compassion on me
It makes me feel like I am touching your divinity
I can feel your divinity expanding in my existence
I happily accept your love-filled blessing
and take this delicate responsibility of nurturing your
fragment within me
I am very grateful to you for this blessing growing within me
I am grateful to you wholeheartedly for this blessing of
motherhood

4. Prayer 4 – Lord of Sun

O Lord of Sun,
Send one the rays of your magnificent divinity within me

23

Shower your magnificence upon me by blessing a new life
within me
Life on the planet is because of you.
Light in the sky is because of you
Shower your blessings on my divine child
Let him always walk on the path enlightened by you
In your light, let him walk towards his life mission
Let your light always be his path of life
Through your light, let his life be pure
Through your light, let his life be magnificent

5. **Prayer 5 – Post-conception**[xiii]

O Lord,
I am very grateful to you for this new life growing within me
I am blossoming with positivity
I am overflowing with love, gratefulness, and enthusiasm
You have given a new meaning to my life
I am aware of every moment
I am doing all the developmental activities for the best
development of my baby
I am happy and I am spreading happiness
I am experiencing your divinity and peace within

6. **Prayer 6 – Pre-conception**

है परमात्मा
है सृष्टि के रचयिता देवो
हमें आपका एक और सुंदर सरजन प्रदान करो
हमें आपकी संवधित शक्तियां
साकार स्वरूप में भेट दो
है ब्रह्मा
आपकी सरजन शक्ति से विभुशीत
आपका बाल स्वरूप हमें प्रदान करो
है विष्णु
आपकी पालन शक्ति के पर्याय:
आप का बाल स्वरूप हमें प्रदान करें
है शिव
हयात संधारक शक्ति के अंश जैसा
कलेसो का नास करें ऐसी शक्ति वाला
बालजीव हमें प्रदान करें

7. Prayer 7 – Post-conception

है ब्रह्माण्ड के देवी देवता
मुझे एक वीर, बुद्धिशाली और
सर्व गुण सम्पन्न बालक प्रदान करो
है प्रभु
मुजे एक साहसी, दयावान, धर्यशील,
दानवीर शिशु प्रधान करो
है प्रभु
मुजे एक विवेकवान, चरित्रवान,
आदर्शों का पालन करने वाला, दिव्य बालक प्रधान करो
मेरा संतान माता पिता और देश का नाम
समग्र विश्व में रोशन करे
ऐसा मुझे आशीर्वाद दो

8. Prayer 8 – Post-conception

है प्रभु
नवजीवन की रचना के हेतू
आपने मुझे पसंद किया
उसके लिए आपका अंतरकरण से शुक्रिया
है ईश्वर
मेरी कोख में जो शिशु पल रहा है
वो आपका ही अंश है
आप मुझे इतना समर्थ देना
जिस्से आपके इस स्वरूप को
आपके ही अनुरूप बना सकु
मेरी कोख से एक श्रेष्ठ आत्मा अवतार हो
ऐसे योग बनाओ
यह श्रेष्ठ आत्मा द्वारा उसके कारियो से
इस जगत का कल्याण हो

DO IT RIGHT

1. One hour and 36 minutes before sunrise is called Brahma Muhurat. During this time, the universe guides us towards our highest potential and positively impacts our minds and bodies.
2. Everything in this universe, whether living or non-living, is made up of energy.
3. Our words, intentions, and thoughts have energy and are potent weapons that can create or destroy anything.
4. Prayer unleashes the highest form of energy. A mother can channel positive energy towards her womb and facilitate healthy fetus development by praying daily.
5. The camphor vapors are anti-viral, anti-bacterial, and anti-fungal. They have a therapeutic effect on the body and the mind.

27

CHAPTER 3
BABY ALBUM

Riya wore a long blue skirt and pink floral blouse with a grey handbag on her left shoulder. She wondered why they were asked to carry a drawing book, sketch pens, and crayons for today's session. She was terrible at drawing. She moved up and down her room anxiously, with crayons in her hands, thinking how bad she was. She thought about her sitar performances at college fests. *Why couldn't drawing be as easy as playing the sitar?* Music connected her with her soul. She shrugged her shoulders and asked Alexa to play Pandit Ravi Shankar's album. She took a deep breath and started getting ready for the session. The sitar music was feeding her soul and easing all her stress. Soon she was relaxed and she left for the session at 4:30 a.m.

All the women were very excited about this unique session. Few even made plans to draw the river, mountains, sunsets and many more.

"Good morning," Ananya greeted Riya chirpily.

It was different today because an ordinarily introvert Ananya seemed talkative. She was gleeful like a baby. After all, she got a chance to be with her first passion - crayons and drawing book, after fifteen long years.

She sensed the uneasiness in Riya and asked, "Hey, what's wrong with you today?"

Riya kept looking at her crayons and drawing book, "I am a little nervous. I am terrible with these."

Ananya laughed and said, "Relax, Riya! We are not giving any exams. We are here to enjoy and the Ancient Guru will take care of everything."

The Ancient Guru walked to the stage surrounding the Banyan tree and greeted everyone, "Good morning."

All the eyes were now on the Ancient Guru.

A woman in the third row wearing a pastel blue saree thanked the Ancient Guru for asking to bring the drawing book. She shared that the very act of just buying these things for herself touched the little child in her, which was buried under her adulthood and responsibilities.

The Ancient Guru smiled and said, "I understand you, my light warrior! We all have been so busy living life according to others' wants and expectations that we have forgotten our true selves. Today is the day of creativity. And not just any creativity; it's for the baby of your dreams."

The Ancient Guru paused to look into everyone's eyes. The energy of the crowd was at a different level today. Their eyes were gleaming.

He thought that the purpose of the session was already served and asked, "How many of you know which attributes and virtues you desire in your baby? I want all of you to close your eyes for a moment and think about it."

The crowd obeyed and there was pin-drop silence. The only sound that could be heard was of rushing cold winds softly kissing the light warriors' skin and chirping birds filling the heart with melody. The smell of the morning dew was tranquilizing their minds and calming them. The soothing sound of the waterfall was making the session meditative as if

29

it was covering up the whole area with a blanket of positivity and blessing these strong and dedicated mothers.

Perfectionist Ananya could quickly think of over twenty qualities because of her strong logical mind. In contrast, Riya just wanted her baby to be happy inside out; and have a friendly and bubbly nature like her.

The Ancient Guru said, "We all know that everything is energy. Our words, thoughts, emotions, and actions set out definite signals to the universe. Depending on what we desire, the universe manifests it. Today in this drawing book, you will draw the whole life of your baby, right from birth to death. We will break it into different sections to vividly picture the baby's life. You need to write what your baby would do at that particular age along with his qualities."

RITUAL #2: Create Your Baby Album And Read It Daily

A petite lady wearing black jeans and a dark green shirt with short hair asked, "Won't this be forcing the life from our perspective on the baby? Shouldn't we let the baby live the life of his own choice?"

"That's a good question, my light warrior!" exclaimed the Ancient Guru. "But, we are not forcing anything on the baby. We are not selecting any profession for him. We are just setting out the intention that he excels in whatever he chooses. In reality, we always guide our children. Don't we force them to eat healthy food, brush their teeth twice a day, or complete their education? Do we give them the liberty to give up their education?

"No," answered the crowd.

"Why?" asked the Ancient Guru. "Because we all want the best life for our children. We know how important education is. That's why we want our children to study. Similarly, during pregnancy, mothers take utmost care of their eating habits for the baby's best development. But they fail to take care of their thoughts and emotions and ignore their spiritual well-being. Through today's activity, I want you all mothers to set out a definite intention on the kind of life you want for your baby and surrender it to the universe."

The Ancient Guru continued, "I will give you the sample statements for every section for more clarity. When you look into history, the mothers knew how their children would be, even before conceiving. We know about Queen Madalsa now. In India, the women were very spiritual and courageous. The whole generation of freedom fighters who were willing to sacrifice their lives for the nation resulted from brave mothers relentlessly willing to end the British rule and free their country."

A lady in her late 30s raised her hand. She asked, "But why these drawing books, Guruji? Why can't we simply list down the qualities?"

The Ancient Guru clapped and answered, "This was a great question. The question for which I had been waiting. If I were to teach you something, you would like to be taught by instructions, or would you prefer the pictorial representations whenever possible?"

"Pictorial representations," all the women shouted in unison.

The women unknowingly got their answers. They looked at each other and started smiling.

The Ancient Guru looked at each one of them and inhaled deeply. He had mastered the breathing techniques through

31

years of practice. He tapped into the abundance of energy primarily through his breath and meditative state of mind.

He said, "That's exactly why we need things of art today. The universe understands our intentions better when we can visualize them and feel them. The more vivid our description, the more we live by it and the more are the chances of them being manifested[xiv]. This is the **'Power of VISUALIZATION'**. This technique has been practiced since time immemorial to fulfill all the desires of humankind[xv]. If all of you agree with this and it touched your heart, you can say AHA."

And the crowd roared with AAHA sound.

The Ancient Guru continued, "Today, you are going to visualize the entire life of your baby. So, paint it with colors, list down all his strengths, quality of life, values, virtues, emotions, and higher purpose and impact on society. Through visualization, you can even attract the physical attributes of your baby. Those who want to attract certain physical attributes can even select their dream baby picture and stick it on the first page of their drawing book. There is nothing wrong with it, but for me, the qualities and virtues matter the most as they would ultimately serve society. So, I have kept the photo activity optional. After you complete your baby album, read it consistently every day throughout your pregnancy journey so that you can visualize the whole life of your baby and manifest it into reality. You can also ask your husbands to contribute to creating the baby album. Let's begin this ritual now. You can have a look at some sample sentences. And you need to complete your baby album today itself. That's your homework for today, in addition to praying daily."

"Sangachadwam."

The Ancient Guru blessed everyone and left.

Ten ladies wearing bright yellow chiffon saree started distributing sample sheets.

BABY ALBUM STATEMENTS

1) Photo of your Dream Baby (Optional)

You can search for the picture of the baby with the physical attributes you desire. It can be the skin complexion, eye color, hair type, etc. Mothers can even search for their favorite celebrity's childhood photo if they desire.

2) Prayer

Chose the prayer with which you are most connected. Pray to the divine and seek his blessings in the form of new life within you. Your prayer must include the qualities you desire in the child and surrender your desires to the divine.

3) Emotional Connection

We will create deeper bonds between the family members and the baby so that he will know the family members right from the womb. He will have deeper bonds with them when he comes into this world. Here you need to go to your family members and ask them what kind of relationship they would like to have with your baby. Write their message in your album with their picture next to their message. You can start with your picture first, then your husband and later the rest of the family members. It is crucial to ensure that you don't use negative terms and write in the present tense.

4) Conception Preparation

You can add this section if you have not conceived yet and are in the pre-pregnancy stage. Mention here all those things you

33

are doing to purify your gametes, body, mind and soul. Read it daily to attract the divine blessings. It will give you the energy to be consistent and bring transformation. Sample statements:

i. I am eating wholesome, nutritious homemade food for you, baby, because I know well that you eat what I eat
ii. I have become an early riser because I know it has tremendous benefits
iii. I am attending Garbh Sanskar classes regularly
iv. I have started reading good books regularly
v. I work-out daily
vi. I meditate daily
vii. I spend some time with nature daily

Pregnant mothers can skip this section in their baby album.

5) Mother's Commitment

We will then move towards what you are doing during pregnancy for the baby's best development. Make your list. The list must have work done on all aspects such as physical, mental, emotional and spiritual. Reading this list consistently will strengthen your commitment to what you decide to do during your pregnancy journey. Some affirmative statements are:

i. I eat tasty sattvic food for your best physical and mental development, baby
ii. I do yoga regularly to increase prana energy within me.
iii. For the best development of your mind, I meditate and do pranayamas daily
iv. I listen to good music for your all-round development
v. I am reading good books regularly
vi. I solve puzzles daily for your best logical development
vii. To feel you within me is the best experience of my life
viii. You are part of my existence
ix. I am enjoying my pregnancy completely

6) Child Birth

We don't want to decide the day and time for the baby's birth. We want the process to be enjoyable for both mother and the baby. During labor, most women are stressed, start shouting, are scared, and crib and send negative emotions to the baby. The day that was supposed to be the best day of your life turns into a nightmare you have dreaded since conception. The day your baby is born is no less than a festival for you. You had been waiting for this day since you got to know about your pregnancy. Yet mothers forget this, and they suffer, and the baby suffers with them too.

Some so-called modern mothers even favor planned caesarean despite knowing its disadvantages. I am not against the surgeries, but they should be resorted to as the last option and not as the first preference. Because of a few misguided professionals and mothers, babies suffer. Their immunity gets compromised, and we have a generation of people with weak immunity and damaged psychology[xvi]. Caesarean doesn't just affect the baby's immunity; it has a profound psychological impact leaving the imprints of insecurity deep down in the baby[xvii].

> **BREAST CRAWL**
>
> Dear light warriors! I strongly recommend you all to opt for breast crawl. The first hour post-delivery is very crucial and your baby needs you the most at that time. Be there for him and keep him as close to you as possible. Several studies suggest that breast crawl deepens the bond between mother and baby, helps in expulsion of placenta, eases breast feeding, reduces postpartum depression, calms the baby and gives him sense of security.

I don't want you, my warriors, to suffer. All of us shall always prefer normal delivery for the best of the baby and the mother.

In this section, mention what you would do to facilitate normal delivery. Sample statements:

i. Baby, you are born on the best day, time and method decided by divine

ii. Natural birth increases your immunity baby

iii. I am regularly going to pregnancy classes for your best growth

iv. I am taking good care of my food, exercise and breathing techniques to facilitate normal vaginal delivery with ease.

v. I am practicing yogic delivery technique in my 9^{yh} month of pregnancy

vi. Baby, you are coming into this world with ease

vii. We are having normal, painless delivery

viii. Baby, you are mentally, physically and emotionally fit and healthy

ix. The best quality and quantity of breastmilk is being produced for your best development.

x. Baby, you can digest the milk with ease and are smiling all the time

xi. Baby, you can suck the milk very easily and are enjoying it

xii. Baby, you are taking enough sleep and loving everything and everyone around you

7) Child's Life

It is the last section of the baby album. Here we will divide your baby's life into various parts and write down the qualities you would like to see in him during that phase of life. Here you will design his entire life and send your blessings to him to live his life to its fullest potential.

The first statement in each section here will be, "According to your age, your physical, mental, emotional and spiritual development is at the best level. Your five senses are getting developed very well along with your 6th sense intuition."

Then the statements will differ depending on the phase of life. Sample Statements are as follows:

I.   0 – 3 Months
   i.   You brought happiness to the lives of everyone in the family
   ii. Everyone loves to spend time with you, baby. You are everyone's favorite
   iii. You love to be with and play with everyone
   iv. Baby loves to take a bath and body massage daily
   v.   You love to listen to the music you had heard when you were in the womb. It takes you into a meditative state
   vi. You feel calm when you spend time with nature
   vii. You are enjoying this beautiful world thoroughly
   viii. Baby loves to see the sky, sleep below the sky, see sunrise, sunsets, moon, stars, trees, leaves, flowers, flying birds and the sea. You are so amazed at seeing them that they bring a different shine to your eyes
   ix. You are full of energy. Baby, you emit radiance
   x.   You have a big smile when you go to sleep and you wake up with that big smile

II.   4 – 6 Months Old
   i.   You are happy with yourself and you are enjoying your own company
   ii. You are always smiling and happy. Because of this, everyone loves to be with and play with you
   iii. You feel satisfaction from within all the time, Baby
   iv. You can express your choice of music very quickly.
   v.   You are very responsive. You show your emotions so well all the time
   vi. You enjoy being close to nature. You love to play in the garden and go to the temple

    vii.   Baby, you have a heart of gold

III.   7 – 9 Months Old
- i. You love to eat sattvic food for your best physical and mental development
- ii. You are happy with all healthy food, and you can digest it easily
- iii. Baby, you respond to music very happily by dancing, manifesting your connection with music
- iv. The teeth eruption process is easy and healthy for you
- v. You have excellent concentration skills, focus and perseverance
- vi. You love everything and everyone around you. You are the epicenter of joy for the people around you
- vii. Baby, you have an innocent face, black eyes, a beautiful smile, and are very joyful. Because of this, your personality is very attractive and mesmerizing. You can influence everyone around you
- viii. You have a very sharing nature, baby. You can share your toys and food with everyone easily
- ix. You have very strong immunity and your digestive system is working very well
- x. You are very patient, calm and composed and you are very balanced
- xi. You are a very cheerful, playful and healthy baby
- xii. Baby, you love to be with nature

IV.   10 – 12 Months Old
- i. You bond with other kids very quickly and you like to play with everyone around
- ii. Your language is pure, clear, respectful, polite, sweet and direct from your heart

iii. You can sing very well and play musical instruments easily
iv. You like to play in a natural environment
v. You can express your needs and requirements very easily
vi. You have respect and compassion for the whole of the natural world
vii. You have a very compelling way of speaking. You can easily influence others through your speech
viii. Your body language is very attractive
ix. You can do yoga easily

V. 1 – 2 Years Old *You are navigating this 'cultural' differences seamlessly*

i. You can understand the feelings and emotions of others easily and you can express your feelings very clearly
ii. You can understand every subject, object, and situation quickly and stay balanced
iii. You are very clear about your emotions
iv. You possess the quality of being just and neutral
v. You are very creative and keep innovating new things with your limited resources. *but earth's vast resource*
vi. You have leadership and management qualities and love to lead in all the roles
vii. You are full of innocence, simplicity and compassion
viii. You love to listen to stories, mantras, shlokas and lullabies and you like to narrate the same to others
ix. You enjoy listening to *& playing* music and doing yoga, *dance & athletics*
x. You can play happily with other kids *& make friends easily*
~~xi.~~ You like to do plantations, take care of plants, visit the zoo and be in the natural environment
xii. You are always full of energy, vigor and confidence
xiii. You are everyone's favorite and they like to play with you and spend their time with you
xiv. You have a very high awareness of your inner and outer world *You speak clearly & attract everyone with your dynamic & charming personality*
You love reading

You love your quiet time, where you read

JUHI SOHAL

You are happy go lucky and independent
self aware

VI.   2 – 3 Years Old

You are curious, a keen observer & a creative thinker

i.   You are very creative and are always busy with your creative activities

ii.   You respect and follow our culture

iii.   You are very independent. You do all your work by yourself

iv.   You like to maintain hygiene. You keep yourself and your surroundings clean

v.   You are very obedient and you respect your elders

vi.   You are very kind at heart and you like to help others

vii.   You like to visit places which are close to nature

viii. You love to chant OM, listen and recite shlokas, do yoga, pranayama, meditation, and prayer daily

You are growing into a strong athlete, a leader, a visionary. You enjoy listening/playing music

VII.   School Period

i.   You follow a *healthy* ayurvedic dincharya

ii.   You like to keep your surroundings and room neat and clean

iii.   You treat younger ones with love and care and elders with respect

iv.   You love to be with nature

v.   You enjoy all sports

vi.   You give your 100 % in all the activities you do

vii.   You compete with yourself and strive to be your best version

viii. You love to do yoga, pranayama, meditation and other exercises

ix.   Your courage and fearlessness are reflected in your actions and attitude

x.   You always live in the present moment

xi.   Baby, you love to go to school. You know school is significant in life. You enjoy learning new things in school *& outside of it*

xii.   Because of your joyful, helpful and sharing nature with a smiling face, you are everyone's favorite in the school

You are blossoming into an influential entrepreneur & leader. You continue to 40 think outside of the box/ & beyond the education system while excel at both

You are navigating your ethnicity & culture & religions well & use it as an advantage. You are growing undeterred & unwan cross a leader

xiii. You love to write stories poems, sing songs and play *loader* musical instruments

xiv. You enjoy learning new languages *& becoming an avid, multiple boy*

xv. You make the atmosphere positive with your powerful aura whenever you go

xvi. You love to read books and you have your library

xvii. You feel content within yourself *with a strong sense of self & directs*

xviii. You are everyone's favorite in the family and everyone loves to spend time with you

xix. Baby, you have been very creative since your birth.

xx. You love to recite Sanskrit shlokas and learn our ancient knowledge

xxi. You earn along with your school and spend it for the betterment of the society

xxii. You are very skillful, and you excel in all extracurricular activities

xxiii. You are full of enthusiasm

xxiv. You have curiosity, Baby. Your soul loves knowledge. You respect and take an interest in knowing new things

xxv. Because of your powerful concentration, observation, desire, memory power and grasping ability, you can learn new skills, things and activities quickly

xxvi. You have a deep, peaceful and relaxing sleep. You sleep in the receptive mode and receive positive energy

You have an amazing ability to make connects across disciplines – arts & sciences, humanities & tech for unparalleled innovation, imagination & genius

VIII. College Life

i. You are getting the best knowledge from your teachers, friends, parents, society, relatives, coaches and nature for your mission in life

ii. You are very modest and humble. You have a righteous and transparent character in society

iii. You like to do the Bhangra *dance & sports* as part of your physical workout in your free time. You are also known for your good sense of humor

iv. You have blossomed spiritually and always stay balanced and focused

41

You are an accomplished student, a successful athlete, a visionary leader, a strong entrepreneur with a clear sense of direction

v. You are the favorite of all professors and you are very popular amongst students at your college

vi. You participate in college activities and lead in most of them

vii. Self-confidence, pure speech, simplicity, sharing, enthusiasm, creativity, charming, leadership and honesty make you a very attractive and influential personality

viii. You have aligned your passion with your profession and you are in your field of interest at the best time

ix. You are meticulous about your eating habits and you prefer to eat food as essential to your body's requirements

x. Yoga, pranayama, meditation and physical fitness is undivided part of your life, amongst other things

xi. You give enough time to your hobbies which feed your soul

You are social, well connected, reach for people - critical to your success with no hesitation

IX. Professional Life

i. You follow ayurvedic dincharya diligently

ii. You earn well and also serve society through your work

iii. You find a perfect balance in your professional and personal life

iv. You always live in the present moment without any regrets about the past and worries about the future

v. Your action matches your words and thoughts. Commitment is your strength

vi. You feel very blessed and you can surrender yourself to the Divine and live a stress-free life

vii. You follow the good deeds of great people who revolutionized the world through their ideas and commitment. Ex. Persistence of Gandhi, the wisdom of Tagore

viii. Honesty, hardworking, just, transparent, grateful, selfless, joyful, friendly, helpful and positive attitude are the factors that contribute to your excellence in your work

ix. Yoga, pranayama, meditation and physical exercises are an inseparable part of your daily routine
x. You live a life full of gratitude
xi. You have perfect social status
xii. You are super-rich and independent
xiii. Apart from professional, internal development is a significant part of your life
xiv. You always admire the beauty and power of nature and strive to be connected to it *You continue to engage in hobbies to feed your soul*

X. Marriage Life

i. All members of our family respect each other and care for the feelings and emotions of each other *You both*
ii. Your life partner is very loving and caring. ~~She~~ keep*s* the whole family together and connected
iii. You and your wife push each other's development and grow economically, socially, physically, emotionally and spiritually
iv. She is full of virtues, morals, positivity and peace-loving
v. You both make a power couple and are an inspiration for many
vi. You have a wonderful and happy married life
vii. You both love each other daily a bit more
viii. We are delighted with you, baby
ix. Our family is the ideal family *We continue to maintain our family trips & ritual & gatherings*

XI. Parenthood

i. You are giving good quality time to your family
ii. You are very good at parenting and you are giving in your best efforts
iii. For your child's best development, you are physically, mentally, socially, emotionally and spiritually at the best of your time
iv. Through stories, kathas, knowledge, experiences, we are contributing to the lives of our grandchildren

v. We enjoy going to gardens, temples, beaches, etc. with our grandchildren

vi. We are delighted with our grandchildren and we are enjoying this phase of life

XII. Grandparenthood
i. At this level, you are enjoying life with your grandchildren
ii. We are on cloud nine and thoroughly enjoying our life with our great-grandchildren
iii. You are very happy and satisfied with the economic, social, spiritual, mental and emotional growth you have achieved in your life
iv. We are all a very happy and big family and feel blessed

Ananya quickly moved her eyes through the sheet and exclaimed, "This is pure genius!". Few eyes turned over her. She patted her forehead with her right palm and started creating her baby album. The instructions also stated that the mother could draw supporting images while giving descriptions such as a tie showing the school period, bubble bathing baby vector, baby clothes, sleeping baby, etc. It was a fun activity.

Ananya loved the game of chess and wanted her baby to know it so that they can play together. She included it in her baby album and drew a king vector from the chess game.

Riya saw the infinity tattoo on Ananya's right wrist while she was drawing. Riya complimented her and they worked on the album together.

Riya exhaled a breath of relief as it wasn't what she thought. There wasn't just drawing involved. She also loved the sample examples but added a few more points to make them more relatable. She quickly searched for the Bollywood actor Hritik Roshan's childhood picture on google and gave the picture to one of the volunteers for print. She recalled how she used to watch the first show of his every movie and sleep with his poster under her pillow in her college days. She wasn't biased towards gender, but since she had a 3-year-old baby girl Navya, her heart desired a baby boy this time. She used to be so obsessed with Hritik Roshan that sometimes Varun would tease her, saying, "Please don't leave me when you get proposed to by Hritik." Riya's cheeks would turn all red, and meekly she would say, "I will leave everything and go with Hritik." She enjoyed this teasing from Varun. But after Navya was born, she almost forgot about her first crush on this superstar and got busy with life. Today, when the Ancient Guru said that even physical attributes could be attracted, a gush of energy ran through her body and she knew what she wanted.

The volunteer came to her with the hard copy of the photo and broke Riya's train of thought. She scanned it and glued it immediately on the first page of her drawing book. Then she worked on the rest of the baby album.

DO IT RIGHT

1. Our words, thoughts, emotions, and actions set out definite signals to the universe. Depending on what we desire, the universe manifests it.
2. The universe understands our intentions better when we can visualize them and feel them.
3. Visualization technique has been practiced since time immemorial to fulfill all the desires of humankind.
4. Through the baby album, a mother can attract the baby of her dreams.

CHAPTER 4
NATURE EVALUATION

A nanya woke up at 4 a.m. and started reading her baby album immediately. The Ancient Guru had instructed that everyone must read the baby album at least once a day with full awareness. He advised to read it after waking up because the mind was fully aware at that time but asked not to be too rigid and the baby album could be read at any time of the day. The most important point was **CONSISTENCY**.

Ananya had a sense of accomplishment as she completed reading her baby album. *This one step was so valuable.* She felt the power equivalent to mother nature. She felt as if she was writing the destiny of her baby. She joined her hands and expressed gratefulness to the Divine for giving her the opportunity to meet the Ancient Guru.

Arjun woke up. He saw the time and looked at Ananya, "Hey, Love! Good morning, started praying already?" Arjun laughed. "Wouldn't you be late for your class?"

Ananya gave him a small peck, saw the clock and rushed to the washroom to get ready.

Ananya managed to reach the class on time. The Ancient Guru was already on the stage under the Banyan tree. She had worn a coffee brown jumpsuit with copper buttons with her rose gold watch perfectly complemented her jumpsuit. Riya waved at her. Ananya grinned and sat beside her.

"Today is a very interesting day. You will get to know about yourself. You will see the real you with all the faces off your skin. Today you will know your truest self."

"Are you all ready?" asked the Ancient Guru.

"Yes," the crowd said in unison.

"Great! Buckle up your belts for this journey of meeting your true self. We will remove all the masks you have been wearing for many years. Please don't be scared, my light warriors! You are not here to judge yourself or anyone else. Your baby's nature depends on your nature. That is why today you will see your most authentic self," the Ancient Guru said.

A woman sitting in the first row wearing a long maroon kurta and palazzo pants raised her hands and asked, "Master, why do we need to know ourselves? How is it connected with our pregnancy?"

The Ancient Guru answered, "My dear, wonderful question! Let me give you an analogy. Have you ever planted a seed? Have you taken care of the sapling and nurtured it so that it can grow into a shrub or a tree? What does a seed need to grow?"

Ananya spoke this time, "Soil, water, compost, air and sunlight."

All eyes were on her now for that crisp answer.

The Ancient Guru responded, "Well answered."

A few women clapped for Ananya.

"Similarly, your baby is the seed and your body is the soil and the food you eat are the nutrients. The growth of your baby will depend on these things. But this is limited to only physical development. What about mental, emotional and spiritual development? Do you remember that African ritual of forgiveness? Similarly, if you bless a dying plant, it will grow back miraculously," the Ancient Guru paused and watched the crowd.

Everyone was listening to the Ancient Guru with the utmost attention. They all got the point now as to why they needed to evaluate themselves.

The Ancient Guru inhaled deeply and said, "Your thoughts, emotions, habits and actions have a direct and profound influence on the fetus. Your emotions are your baby's emotions; your thoughts are his thoughts; your senses are his senses. Do you get it now? That is why it's important to know the real you. You need to know your thoughts, virtues and good qualities so that you can strengthen your strong points and **more importantly, minimize your weakness and negative qualities.**"

 RITUAL #3: Know Your Most Authentic Self

"Further, the fruits of the tree depend on the seeds. You cannot expect a neem tree to fetch mango fruits no matter how much you pray for it. That's the law of nature. Your prayers are your desires. The baby album is your desire. But, desire alone doesn't change anything. Actions change things. Imagine you pray to God each day to make you fit. You pray wholeheartedly but do nothing towards it. Would anything change?"

Everyone laughed.

"It's the same with your baby, my light warriors. This evaluation is the most important part of this book. How your baby will be depends on this evaluation. But do remember, for eating mangoes, you need to plant mango seeds. It would be best if you were ready to do the work. If you aren't willing to work on yourself, then read no further. Garbh Sanskar isn't for you if you are unwilling to change yourself; work on yourself and become your best version. **Garbh Sanskar is not easy but it's the right thing to do.** I call you warriors for a reason. Changing oneself is one of the most difficult things on this planet. But, today, you have a chance to do it for yourself, your family and most importantly, for your baby. To attract the baby of your dreams, you have to live this knowledge. Match your frequency to the frequency of the universe. Then the miracles will happen and you will give birth to a soul which is bound to bring revolution in the society and make this world a better place."

All the eyes sparkled up. Riya told herself *I am ready to do whatever it takes for the best development of my baby.* She was munching some soaked almonds today. Hunger pangs were troubling her more these days with the growing needs of the baby.

"We all want the best baby, but are we the best?" asked the Ancient Guru. "Please raise your hands whoever thinks they are the best and there is no scope for improvement."

No one raised their hands.

"No one, right? Because we all know that we can improve. Raise your hands if you think you can improve," directed the Ancient Guru.

Everyone raised their hands. The wave of positivity was spread across the park. It wasn't just a simple act of raising a hand. It was about their resolution, determination, and commitment to change themselves, to give away the old habits that pull them down, do whatever it takes for the best development of their baby, and make this world a better place to live. They were no longer selfish. Selfish people cannot change themselves. It's only when one works for the higher cause that one can change oneself. They were now ready. They had now become the light warriors in the truest sense.

"The science of Garbh Sanskar is all about maximizing your positives and minimizing your negatives. Through Garbh Sanskar, you will work for the baby's best physical, mental, emotional and spiritual development. You will be able to give birth to a genius baby and serve society," said the Ancient Guru.

Garbh Sanskar = Maximizing Positives + Minimizing Negatives

The Ancient Guru asked his volunteers to distribute the nature evaluation sheet. Ananya grabbed her off-white handbag tightly. She closed her eyes and focused on her breathing. She had always been scared of judgments. Today with the evaluation, she felt like it was a judgment day for her. She had strived for perfection throughout her life, but her pursuit had stolen happiness from her inner being. In her quest for perfection, she lost her inner child. She held the nature sheet, prayed to the Divine and hoped for the best.

The Ancient Guru was watching everyone closely. His eyes sensed the tension and uneasiness on many faces. He got up from his wooden chair and looked at the crowd, making eye contact with every mother, "This test isn't the question of life and death, my warriors. Take it easy. Does anyone of you want to ask me anything before we start?"

Ananya raised her hand and asked, "Master, what if we fail? what if we are not perfect?"

51

The Ancient Guru smiled and answered, "There is nothing like a failure. Every failure is great learning. The difference between a successful person and an unsuccessful person is the number of times they have tried. A successful person has failed more times than an unsuccessful person has ever tried. And here you are just meeting your true self with whom you have been living for years. Isn't it interesting?"

"You will know about your strong and weak points, so why worry? There is no such thing as perfection. All of us are flawed. Perfection is a myth. It's different for different people. For you, something might be perfect but for me, it might not be. Also, tell me, who defines it? Running after perfection is a perfect way to steal happiness from our inner self. Perfection stresses out our minds, it doesn't let the mind rest and the end result is also not worth it."

Ananya had tears in her eyes. *I have spent my whole life running behind perfection.*

"All our lives, we are busy writing the script for others[xviii]. We do this very often, especially with our loved ones. We say that that person should do it, my relative must do that, my husband should behave this way and so forth. We do this and start living under the illusion that we are perfect ourselves."

This hit Riya hard. She found herself often trying to control Varun's life. She would fail each time and get frustrated at not being able to change him at all.

"We waste our time and energy in our efforts to change others. But has anyone ever been successful? Please raise your hands if anyone of you has been successful and we will have a session with her," the Ancient Guru laughed.

The crowd laughed along and the park was filled with laughter.

"So, what's the point in wasting our time and energy towards something which cannot happen?" asked the Ancient Guru.

Few women nodded. The eyes of some women widened at this new revelation.

"The only person we can change is ourselves. And trust me it's a lot easier. You can change only one person, i.e., YOU, but sadly, we never think that way. We live under the illusion that we are the best. We always think the problem is with others and not with us. For example, after two days of marriage, the wet towel was on the bed and after two years, the wet towel still lies on the bed. Has anything changed despite asking to change for 400 days?"

A few women from the crowd laughed out loudly. They could really connect with the example. Ananya grinned.

"So, let's break that illusion today. We might have complaints about so many people. Similarly, so many people might have complaints about us too," said the Ancient Guru.

"Children are the reflection of their parents. So, through this evaluation, we will make the best reflection."

Ananya's eyes sparkled again. She wondered how the Ancient Guru knew so much. She felt lighter in her heart. *I will become a better version of myself. It was time for Ananya 2.0.*

The Ancient Guru continued, "Let's look into how the brain works for more clarity. We have two minds – the conscious mind and the subconscious mind. The former does all the decision making while the latter has unlimited potential."

CONSCIOUS MIND

- Dominant

- Diplomat

- Limited
  Potential

- Decision
  Making

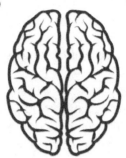

SUBCONSCIOUS MIND

- Submissive

- Truthful

- Unlimited
  Potential

- Intuitive

B R A I N

"While taking decisions, there is a little voice from our subconscious mind which speaks to us. Sometimes, we listen to it but we mostly ignore it and follow our conscious mind. If things don't go as planned, then we think that the little voice was right. The first answer to all your questions comes from the subconscious mind[xix]."

"In this nature evaluation, you need to answer from the subconscious mind and not your conscious mind because if your conscious mind answers the questions, everyone will get a 50+ score. To answer from your subconscious mind, listen to your first instinct – inner voice and avoid the explanations given by your conscious mind because that will defeat the purpose of the evaluation, which is the diagnosis and knowing your true self," suggested the Ancient Guru.

The crowd nodded.

Ananya realized that she had ignored her subconscious mind most of the time. All the situations in which she ignored the subconscious mind came before her eyes and she could see how she could have made better choices in the past.

"So, how should you answer the questions? Are you excited to know?" asked the Ancient Guru.

"Yes!" said the crowd.

"All right! There are 12 questions and each question has a scale of 1 to 5. I will give you five different situations for each question and whenever the situation connects with your inner self, you must circle the answer. Please don't wait to listen to all the situations. Because if you do then you will answer from your conscious mind. Whenever I say a situation and it connects with you, forget everything else and circle the answer. You won't connect with every situation. You would connect with only what you actually are."

"For example, if I say 'all of you must behave politely with your mother-in-law'. Those who are already behaving politely won't be bothered but those who are behaving rudely will definitely be affected by this statement. The statement will pinch them and their mind will start justifying their behavior. In this manner, you will get to know your real self. Let's take another example. Suppose I say 'don't steal today'. Most of us won't be affected by this statement because we don't steal. But if I say 'don't get angry' today, probably 90% of the women present here would be affected. Botherations come only when they show us the real self, overcoming the dominance of the conscious mind. Here, marks don't matter. All of you are equal. Honest evaluation is a must to become your best version. We all have time to improve. But if we don't get the correct diagnosis, then there can be no improvement."

The Ancient Guru continued, "Please don't think about your friends and partners while answering this test. This test isn't about them. Their score doesn't matter."

The crowd chuckled. Riya repeated this to herself. *I should stop writing script for Varun's life.*

"Most women think about their husbands while answering this test. This test is just for you and not for him. For example, if you have a fever, it's you who needs to get the blood test done and not your husband. If you want, we can arrange a test for husbands in another class. But today, at this moment, this test is just for you and your baby. Be here, give your 100 percent; be honest and get ready to meet the real you. So, hereby I invite you all to take up this resolution to serve the society through your motherhood and become your best version," said the Ancient Guru.

"Let's begin. You can see the evaluation sheet. There are 12 questions and each of the questions carries 5 points. And there is a scale from 1-5. After each question, I will give an example so that you can understand it better and give yourself points from 1 - 5 and in the end, we will sum them up. During pregnancy, you should strive for 50+ points. But if you get less, don't get disheartened and we will work on the weak areas."

EVALUATION SHEET

1	I get angry again and again	1 2 3 4 5	I never get angry
2	I am always lazy	1 2 3 4 5	I am never lazy.
3	I always think about myself first	1 2 3 4 5	I always think about others first
4	I am attached to materialistic things	1 2 3 4 5	I am attached to people
5	I get jealous of others easily	1 2 3 4 5	I am happy with others' happiness
6	There is a lack of vigor in my life	1 2 3 4 5	My life is full of vigor
7	There is a constant fear in my life	1 2 3 4 5	There is no fear in my life
8	I cannot trust anyone	1 2 3 4 5	I can trust everyone easily
9	I am not affected by others' pain	1 2 3 4 5	I am easily affected by others' pain
10	I am not grateful for anything in my life	1 2 3 4 5	I am grateful for everything in my life
11	I am not an art lover	1 2 3 4 5	I am an art lover
12	There is no importance of inner development in my life	1 2 3 4 5	Inner development is a crucial part of my life

"Let's look into the various examples to answer through your subconscious mind, have the correct diagnosis, and meet your most authentic self," said the Ancient Guru.

Q.1. ANGER

1 - If you get angry again and again, think no further; you are at No1. People at No1 have no control over their anger. They are constantly irritated by something or the other.

2 – If you get angry only when you commit any mistake, you are at No2.

3 – If you get angry only at others' fault, then you can circle No3.

4 – It doesn't matter to you who is at fault. If you get angry only when a significant loss is incurred, you are at No4.

Ex. You gave your favorite dress to your cousin sister. She had a three-year-old baby and by mistake, the baby spilled ink on your dress. You didn't get angry because it was a small loss. But if you get mad, then you are at No3.

5 – People at No.5 understand the situation and never get angry. The loss, big or small and who commits the mistake is irrelevant. They are untouched by trivial matters.

Ex. Your best friend borrowed your car. He parked it inside his building campus in roofless parking. Renovations were taking place on the 9th floor on the side where the car was parked. A mishap occurred and an iron rod fell from the 9th floor on the car and the windshield broke. Put yourself in this example and see what you would do. If you could understand the situation and stay calm, you are at No5.

These situations are just for reference. You can think of situations in your life and how you would behave and circle the points accordingly.

Q.2. LAZINESS

Here, we are talking about laziness in nature. Laziness isn't just about sleeping the whole day. Sleeping is just a tiny manifestation of laziness in some people. But it's something subtler and more rooted in our nature. We are talking about active laziness. You will also learn which chakra is associated with laziness as we progress further.

1 – People at No1 are procrastinators. These people will not do anything unless there is a considerable loss.

Ex. You know that you are overweight and should be working out, but if you don't do anything about it, you are at No1.

I took this example because it's relatable to most people.

Ex2. You have been prescribed multi-vitamins but you keep forgetting and someone has to remind you to take meds constantly; you are at No1.

2 – If you do what's easy and ignore what's difficult, then you are at No2.

Ex. You were struggling with conception and got your tests done. The doctor suggested you to reduce your abdominal fat and take vitamin tablets. You take the medicines every day but don't work out because taking meds is easy and working out is hard, then you are at No2.

3 – People who will do all the work but only when it becomes urgent and important.

59

Ex. You have a presentation at your office on Saturday that you knew a week before. But, you sit to make the presentation at the last moment under high stress.

Ex2. Now you know about the Baby Album. But how many of you have already started working on it? Most women start their baby album only after they are pregnant and half of them don't even complete it.

4 – These people do all the routine work. They don't crib and leave things for the last moment, but they don't have time for their hobbies and developmental activities. They are happy with the regular flow of life and don't want to devote time to self-development and hobbies.

5 – There is no laziness in the life of people at No5. They are ready to do any activity.

Ex. Many of you might be working in the corporate sector. You have to go to the office at 10 a.m. and come back at 8 p.m. If you wanted to learn guitar and enrol for the 6 a.m. class, then you are at No5. But if you ignore your hobbies, you are at No4.

Q.3. SELFISHNESS
---

1 – If you never make any compromise for anyone, not even for your husband and baby, then you are at No1.

Ex. You and your husband have divided your time for work and leisure. You have booked an appointment for a haircut in your leisure time, but it's nothing urgent. Your husband has an urgent meeting and requests you to postpone your appointment and look after the kids. If you don't cancel your salon appointment and help your husband, you are at No1.

2 – If you can make compromises, but only for your husband and children, you are at No2.

Ex. In the above situation, if you would cancel your salon appointment but only for your husband and children, then you are at No2.

3 – If you can compromise for anyone in your whole family, you are at No3.

4 – People at No4 will think about others – their relatives, neighbors and friends but wouldn't bear any personal loss. They can help as long as they don't incur any loss. To that extent, they can make compromises.

Ex. Your neighbor has a function at her home. She plans to cook food for 100 guests and was searching for another gas stove. You had a spare gas stove. If you give it to her, then you are at No4. If you don't, then you are at No3.

5 – Some people can bear the slight personal loss for the more significant benefit of someone else. If you can do it, then you are at No5.

Q.4. MATERIALISM

1 - People at No1 are very attached to worldly things. They cannot see anything beyond materialistic things. According to the circumstances, their mood changes frequently. If you think you are extremely moody or people believe that you are grumpy and should check your mood before talking to you, you can circle No1.

Ex. You went to a café to meet your friends. You wanted to have your favorite pasta, but it wasn't available. If your mood is completely ruined by it, you are at No1.

2 – If your happiness is dependent on worldly things and not on people, then you are at No2. For people at No2, things

matter a lot. They are not moody but they are adamant. For women, it's mostly regarding their clothes and ornaments.

Ex. If you can't share your clothes with anyone, including your family members, then you are at No2.

3 – Both people and things are essential for these people. But when it comes to choosing between them, the choice is always the worldly things.

Ex. You love your family and relatives, but you can't leave things. It has been two years since your wedding and your cousin's wedding is in 3 months. Due to COVID, their financial situation is not good and you are requested to give your bridal wear for her wedding. But you are very attached to the dress and refuse to give it to her even though you won't wear it again. You are at No3.

4 – It's the reverse of No3 here. Both people and things are important for these people. But when it comes to choosing between them, they will always select people.

Ex. If you give your bridal wear to your cousin in the above example, you are at No4.

5 – Some people are always happy. There is no sense of ownership amongst them. They are not attached to things. If the quality of things doesn't matter to you, if you are okay with living in a tent or using any mobile phone, you are at No5.

Q.5. JEALOUSY

---

1 – These people want an exclusive copy of everything. Exclusivity matters more to them than their likes and dislikes. They enjoy possessions that are unique and rare.

Ex. While going to a function you think your dress should be the best and no one should wear similar clothing or look better than you, then you are at No1

2 – You are okay with others possessing good things; if your things are good, then you can circle No2. You react when others' possessions are better than your possessions.

Ex. You wear your favorite jumpsuit to the party. Your best friend is also wearing a jumpsuit. But her jumpsuit is better than yours and your friends compliment her more. Your mood is completely off and you leave the party. You are at No2

3 – If your relatives and peers have better possessions than you, you don't react but it bothers you; you can circle No3. You keep thinking about it and wish for better possessions.

Ex. In the above situation, you don't leave the party, but you ask from where she bought the dress and kept thinking that you would go to that shop and buy clothes for the next party, you are at No3.

4 – If you can remain neutral towards others' possessions, then you are at No4. It doesn't matter to you what others possess or what you possess. There is no comparison. You don't care about possessions.

Ex. You have a decent phone and your friend possesses the best phone in the market. It doesn't affect you. If you are neutral, then you can circle No4.

5 – If you can be genuinely happy for others' possessions, you are at No5. If you can be comfortable in others' happiness, you can circle No5. It's challenging to do, but you will be very happy and peaceful if you do this.

63

Ex. In most marriages, women are busy criticizing others' clothing. It's a rare sight to see women complimenting other women truly and not just for the sake of it.

Ex2. In the above situation, if you can be truly happy for your friend and compliment his/her phone without feeling any jealousy, then you are at No5.

There is a beautiful quote by Zen Shin.

"A flower does not think of competing to the flower next to it. It just blooms."

Amazing right? A flower doesn't lose its beauty if it compliments another flower. Your beauty doesn't diminish on complimenting your friends, family and even strangers.

Q.6. VIGOR

Before seeing the examples, let's understand vigor first. Vigor means enthusiasm. When you have positive energy to do your routine tasks and hobbies, you have vigor in life. A complete absence of vigor is depression, which includes sitting idle, not talking to anyone, or thoughts of committing suicide in extreme cases. So, lack of vigor means having no interest and enthusiasm in anything.

1 –People at No1 share even good news in a normal tone. They are not excited about anything in life.

Ex. Your brother got admission to IIT and you shared it in your normal tone with no happiness or excitement; you can circle No1.

Ex2. You were planning to conceive, but you couldn't for the last three years and one day, the pregnancy strip had two lines. There was no change in your mood. There was no excitement or happiness within you. If you shared it with your family just like you share the daily menu, you are at No1.

2 – People at No2 are not enthusiastic in routine life. But if there is any marriage, party, festival, or surprise, it fills you up with energy; you are at No2. I call it **Induced Vigor (IV)**. Here your energy is dependent on others. When an atmosphere of enthusiasm is created, you feel vigor in life. On the rest of the days, you do your routine work with boredom.

Ex. Your husband gives you money for shopping. You were very happy as it was unexpected and there was no occasion. That is material-induced vigor.

3 – Most working women crib over the household work and find it burdensome. If you can do the routine work with enthusiasm, you are at No3.

Ex. In the Mission Mangal movie, Vidhya Balan was very involved in her household chores and equally enjoyed her professional work. If you can enjoy both, you can circle No3.

4 – If you have enthusiasm for your self-developmental activities, for your hobbies, for doing work for anyone along with your routine work, then you can circle No4. These happy people make time for their hobbies.

5 – People at No5 are enthusiastic about anything and everything. They don't have any likes or dislikes and enjoy every kind of work. Participation in every activity is their nature. They are always happy. They are untouched by people and situations.

Ex. You plan to watch a movie at your home with your two other friends. They couldn't turn up at the very last moment for some reason. If you can remain untouched and still enjoy watching the movie as planned, you are at No5.

Q.7. FEAR

Being scared of darkness, insects, height, etc., are very trivial fears. Here we aren't talking about them. We are talking about the fears which reside in our nature. We will analyze our deepest fears. The fears that live in the depths of our hearts.

1 – These people are *scared of change*. There is nothing new in their life. If you are afraid to meet new people, try a new dish in a restaurant, or go to a new place for a holiday, then you are at No1. People at No1 dine at the same restaurants, order the same food, buy from the same shops, etc. They dislike changes.

2 – People at No2 take steps to change things but are always scared of failure. The negative thoughts keep running in their minds.
Ex. You try to cook a new dish at home. Thoughts of it not being cooked well keeps your mind engaged.

Ex2. You bake cakes and pastries very well. All your friends and relatives love it. They encourage you to start a bakery business. You agree and begin your business from home but are constantly worried about failure; then you are at No2.

3 – If you don't have any opposing thoughts while starting something new, then you are at No3. You are optimistic about doing new things in your comfort level. You aren't scared of change.

Ex. After your bakery business from home, you open your bakery store in a commercial complex.

4 – You are open to new things outside your comfort level to a certain extent. You are not scared of unknown places. If you are open to growth, you can circle No4.

Ex. You open a chain of a bakery shops in another city. But it has certain limitations. For example, you can't open a shop outside your state or country. You are scared to open your shop outside India.

5 – These people are confident in every aspect of life. There is no fear in their life. They can talk with anyone and do anything without hesitation. They never have any excuses or boundaries. They are not affected by the results.

Ex. Opening bakery shops across the globe.

Q.8. TRUST

Here we will evaluate your ability to trust others and not the other person's trustworthiness. Believe that the other person is trustworthy and reflect upon your actions.

1 – If you can't trust anyone, not even your husband and baby, you are at No1.

Ex. You cannot eat when your husband feeds you if you are blindfolded. If you need to see what he is feeding you, you are at No1.

2 – If you can only trust your family members, you are at No2. But you can't leave things entirely on them. Your mind is constantly engaged on whether they will do it correctly or not and you keep giving reminders.

Ex. You have called for an event planner for your baby's first birthday. Your husband takes care of decoration while you manage the clothes and the food. But you constantly check whether the decoration is being done perfectly or not.

3 –People at No3 can trust family members and relatives.

Ex. In the above situation, if you don't give instructions on decoration and trust that your husband will get it done correctly, you are at No3.

4 – If you can trust unknown people with non-risky work, you are here.

Ex. You recently shifted your home. Your old salon is now very far from your new home. You go and try a new salon. A bad haircut isn't that risky, so if you go for it, then you can circle No4.

5 – These people can trust unknown people even for risky work.

Ex. You were traveling on the outskirts of the city and your car broke down. After 30 minutes of walking, you come across a mechanic. He said you need to leave the car and he would deliver it to your house the next day. The mechanic was unknown to you. If you can't trust him, you are at No4. But if you can trust the unknown mechanic with your car, you are at No5.

Q.9. EMPATHY

Here it's not about being sad for someone. Empathy means understanding the sorrows and emotions of others. Putting yourself in their shoes and then taking steps to ease their pain. It's not about just feeling sorry for them; it's much more than that.

1 – You aren't an empath. You cannot feel the misery of anyone, not even your husband and baby.

2 – You empathize with your husband and baby but no one else. If you can't empathize with anyone else's sufferings and pains, you are at No2.

68

Ex. A 5-year-old baby in your building is badly fractured. You are untouched by the incident.

3 – You have empathy towards your family and society members.

Ex. In the above situation, you can feel the pain of that baby's parents and ask about his health and cook food for them.

4 – If you have empathy towards a particular community, all the people you know, or for people of your city, then you are at No4.

5 – If you empathize with anyone in this world, you are at No5. There is no differentiation within you; you can feel the pain of everything and everyone, including animals and birds. You are always ready to ease others' pain.

Ex. You saw an injured dog while driving. You stop and take the dog to the vet; then you are at No5. If you do it because you are a dog lover, you are at No4, but if you can genuinely feel the pain of animals, you can circle No5.

Ex2. You are at a park. You see a couple. The lady is crying and the man is trying to console her. You knew reiki. You go there and bless the lady even though she is a stranger.

Q.10. GRATITUDE

Gratitude is being thankful for who you are, what you have, and where you are in life. It includes recognizing that you got the chance to be on this planet Earth as a human, which is no less than a miracle. You acknowledge that you are alive today and appreciate people and things in your life.

1 – You aren't grateful for anything in life. You can't find miracles in anything and feel that you have always got less than what you deserve.

2 – You are grateful but only for big surprises.

Ex. You got a surprise holiday to Singapore from your in-laws on your 5th wedding anniversary. You were very happy and grateful to them. But you aren't thankful for small things like your husband packing a lunch box for your baby or your father-in-law (FIL) bringing fruits home.

3 – If you are grateful for small things in life, if you can find happiness in trivial things, you are at No3. But your gratitude is limited to items only and not for the people. You take people for granted and don't value them.

Ex. In the above situation, if you are grateful to your husband and FIL for the small things they do for the family, then you are at No3.

4 – These people are grateful for things and people both. They understand that they are on this planet by divine miracle and appreciate people and things in their lives. But these people are not grateful for failures.

5 – If you can be grateful for anything and everything in life; for your every failure, every success, every learning, every person - whether good or bad, every experience, every holiday, every meal, your clothes, your education, your emotions, then you are at No5. These people are full of gratitude. Everything is considered a blessing by these people. There is nothing good or bad for them. They take every experience positively, live in gratitude and feel the miracles happening every moment.

Q.11. ART LOVER

We all know the various art forms like dance, painting, sketching, playing musical instruments, singing, knitting, crafts, etc. Let's see how much art we have in our lives.

1 – If you don't have any art in your life, then you are at No1.

2 – If you do art only as part of your profession, you are at No2.

Ex. If you are a dancer or drawing teacher, you are at No2 because you perform art as the means of your livelihood.

3 – If you are involved in art as your hobby, then you are here.

Ex. Every Sunday, you paint because you love to paint. But you aren't involved in other arts.

4 – You like to learn new art if the time permits.

Ex. You will only go to a morning drawing class if someone prepares breakfast for you.

5 – You enjoy and appreciate all the art. You are passionate about learning new things; you make time for them. Your pursuit of learning new art doesn't depend on circumstances and people.

Ex. In the above situation, if you wake up early and prepare your breakfast and go to drawing or music class, then you are at No5.

71

Q.12. INNER DEVELOPMENT

Everyone in this world works on physical well-being. Everyone takes a bath, brushes their teeth and combs their hair. These are basics for physical well-being. But very few people know about cleansing their body at a subtle level - cleansing their mind, thoughts, habits, and emotions. We will see how aware we are on this self-cleansing and healing journey.

1 – You don't know anything about inner cleansing. The term self-development doesn't exist in your life.

2 – You know about self-development, but you always procrastinate.

Ex. An ayurvedic doctor told you to wake up before sunrise for indigestion issues. You always decide to wake up early, but you can't do it. But at least you are aware of the inner cleansing and think about doing something. But the intention falls short of actions and commitment.

3 – You do the subtle developmental activities but only under external pressure and in your comfort. You have several ifs and buts before doing the healing work.

Ex. Your husband motivates you to do yoga with him in the morning. You agree but put a condition that you won't be able to make breakfast and hire the cook for preparing breakfast.

4 – You are involved in self-developmental activities. Self-development is an essential part of your life. You are aware of it and follow it consistently. Still, you drop it in case of work pressure, festivals, or other emergencies. Those activities are the first to get off your list in a time crunch.

Ex. You have Diwali puja at your home. Your skip your yoga and meditation practice for two days.

Ex2. You are on vacation to the Maldives. You don't do any self-development work there.

5 – These people never compromise. Unless they are hospitalized, they never skip or miss their inner cleansing. They know that self-development activities are as important as eating food and sleeping.

Ex. You don't drop inner cleansing when you are on holiday or have a function at home. Like most people don't skip brushing their teeth and bathing, they don't miss their inner developmental activities. Some people wake up at 4 a.m. to do their inner healing during functions or festivals. They are very well aware of its importance and never consider it subordinate to physical cleansing.

These situations are just for reference. You can think of situations in your life and how you would behave and circle the points accordingly.

"Our evaluation ends here," said the Ancient Guru. "Don't forget to put the date and marks. Just sum up the numbers you have circled and you will get your marks."

Ananya scored just 27 out of 60. She was upset. She was afraid of not performing well and that is exactly what had happened. Riya fetched 38 points due to her bubbly and friendly nature. She accepted everyone and was okay with most things and people.

Ananya, on the other hand, was very demanding. She sought perfection in everything, which caused stress and unhappiness in her life.

Riya noticed the unhappiness on Ananya's face while she was writing her score. She patted her back and consoled, "Ananya, it's okay. It's just the beginning."

73

Ananya nodded.

"Remember that the Ancient Guru had said in the introductory session that more than 2,50,000 cells of the baby are developing every minute. So, don't stress out. All of us will improve and become our best versions surely under his guidance. If you take it negatively, then it defeats the whole purpose, right?" encouraged Riya.

Ananya hugged her, "I wish I had a sister like you. Thank you so much for supporting me."

Ananya was a single child and had suffered a lot during her childhood. Arjun was the only light of her life. And now, with the help of the Ancient Guru, she was attracting more positivity in her life. Ananya felt determined to work on her weak areas and strengthen her strong areas.

The Ancient Guru asked, "Has everyone completed their evaluation?"

"Yes!" replied the crowd.

"How are the marks? Disappointing?" asked the Ancient Guru.

The crowd made a "Hmmm" sound.

"I would recommend you to repeat this evaluation every month. If you repeat this evaluation, you will know about your progress. Several mothers have improved their scores from the 30s to 50s. But there is another side to this. The score can go down too if you don't live this knowledge and remain disconnected. That is why it's crucial to be with like-minded people. Your community will always have the power to influence you without you even noticing it. If you disconnect, the other forces will start having their influence over you and you will lose the miracle chance for the baby's best development. The marks are not important. What's most important is your awareness of where you stand and where you should be. This is what the test is all about. Now the next step after diagnosis is **IMPLEMENTATION**," explained the Ancient Guru.

Ananya raised her hand and asked, "How can we improve ourselves, Master?"

"It has already been revealed to you, my warriors. Living this knowledge will tremendously impact you and eventually reflect in your score. It's not just your score that changes, but you too change inside out; your thoughts, habits and behavior change. Improvement is not just on paper here. It's the kind of improvement that everyone can notice. But there is a difference between knowing and living the knowledge."

"I will give you a simple example. You see someone asking for directions to a particular location. You know the route, but you don't help unless asked. That is just knowing. Living the knowledge is when you are ready to help anyone at any time. It is the same with every emotion and every quality. Start applying this knowledge. If you can't live it, it won't be imbibed in your baby." *[Reading this book won't help to inculcate the qualities in your baby. This book is just the map. You need to live these rituals for your baby's best development]*

"Let me give you another example. You want to travel to Delhi and ask your best friend to guide you. She gives you the route and details about the trains and their timings. But she can't travel on your behalf. You have to travel on your own. Similarly, you have to go through this **process of transformation**. No one else can do it for you."

The Ancient Guru paused to let the warriors absorb what he had said.

75

Riya and Ananya's eyes were fixed on the Guru just like everyone else without blinking.

"By just attending this session, you won't get your dream baby. You have to live this knowledge every single day. You have to show up to your rituals for your baby. Your baby is your reflection. He will be a magnified version of what you are. If you break small rules, he might break bigger rules. If you tell small lies and expect the baby to be truthful, that is not fair. And he can tell bigger lies too. The baby will learn that it's okay to lie. The baby won't differentiate between a small lie and a big lie. Being untruthful, disloyal, undisciplined and ungrateful and expecting truthfulness, loyalty, discipline, and gratefulness from the baby will be unjust to the baby. If you want these qualities in your baby, start living them this very moment. All I am saying is to expect what you are from the baby. If you are positive, he will be positive 1000x. But, if you are negative and you expect him to be positive, that's futile."

The Ancient Guru continued, "Always remember what Lord Krishna said in Bhagavad Gita Chapter Two Verse Forty-Seven[xx]:"

कर्मण्येवाधिकारस्ते मा फलेषु कदाचन ।

मा कर्मफलहेतुर्भूर्मा ते सङ्गोऽस्त्वकर्मणि । ।

"It means that the only thing in your hands is to give your 100%. You aren't entitled to the fruits of your actions[xxi]. So, don't get attached to the results. Just perform your duty with full faith and leave the results on the Divine[xxii]."

"Surrender your efforts. You will feel light, and the community will give you the energy to bring massive changes in your life for your baby's best development. All the best, my light warriors!"

"Sangachadwam."

The Ancient Guru joined his hands, blessed everyone and left.

DO IT RIGHT

1. Your thoughts, emotions, habits and actions have a direct and profound influence on the fetus. Your emotions are your baby's emotions; your thoughts are his thoughts; your senses are his senses.
2. To attract the baby of your dreams, you have to live this knowledge. Match your frequency to the frequency of the universe and then the miracles will happen.
3. The science of Garbh Sanskar is all about maximizing your positives and minimizing your negatives.
4. Through Garbh Sanskar, you will work for the baby's best physical, mental, emotional and spiritual development.
5. Stop writing the script for others' lives, especially of our loved ones. By dictating other's life, we get the illusion that we are perfect.
6. The only person we can change is ourselves.
7. We have two minds – the conscious mind and the subconscious mind. The former does all the decision-making while the latter has unlimited potential.
8. The first answer to our questions comes from the subconscious mind.
9. Botherations come only when they show us the authentic self, overcoming the dominance of the conscious mind.
10. Honest evaluation is a must to become your best version. But if you don't get the correct diagnosis, there can be no improvement.
11. You cannot control everything. So here is the key - give your 100% and trust the Divine.
12. Be in a like-minded community. You will feel motivated, relaxed and free.

CHAPTER 5
HEALTHY EATING

Ananya woke up at 4 a.m. and read her baby album. She was wearing her pink teddy tee and shorts with rabbit slippers. She always loved these cute things. Arjun often made fun of her saying; he will now have to take care of two babies. "Baby will steal your slippers," he used to tease Ananya. And she would blush.

Arjun heard the noise of pages in the stillness of the night. He cracked open his eyes, saw Ananya and placed his head on her lap. Ananya caressed his hair and continued reading the baby album. Later she went to the bathroom to get ready for the class.

While leaving, she kissed Arjun on his cheeks while he was still lying on the bed. He wished her all the best.

Today, Ananya reached the park a little early. She sat on the swing near the waterfall by the stream. She was enjoying the cool breeze playing with her loosely tied hair. Suddenly, she felt like something was moving around her. She looked around and saw a swan. She smiled. Soon few more swans came and she enjoyed watching them.

Some women also joined her and watched the swans. It filled them with joy.

Soon more crowd gathered and the Ancient Guru also arrived.

Riya called Ananya and they all settled down.

The Ancient Guru went to the stage and greeted everyone. "Today's topic will interest you all. It will be a very interactive session. You might know some things and might wish to add a few more. Can you guess today's topic?"

A woman in the fifth row wearing a big hat answered, "Is it sleep?"

A woman from the first row answered, "Lifestyle?"

Some other answers were physiological changes, mind management, baby health, etc.

The Ancient Guru enjoyed the varied answers. After the crowd stopped answering, he said, "Your guesses were interesting, but today, we will talk about healthy eating."

"Ooooooooooo," said the crowd.

That was easy. Why couldn't I think of it earlier? Ananya thought.

"Why do we eat food?" asked the Ancient Guru.

Riya answered, "Because we feel hungry."

Few women laughed at her answer.

Some other answers were staying fit, staying healthy, for nutrients, etc.

The Ancient Guru continued, "We eat food for energy. Our body needs nutrients for optimal functioning. Ayurveda divides food into three categories - **Sattvic, Rajasic** and **Tamasic.**[xxiii]"

"One should have the highest proportion of sattvic food with some rajasic food and very little tamasic food in one's diet. But

80

during motherhood, you must be more cautious about what you eat as your baby develops taste buds according to your diet. That will ultimately become his choice in the future. You can sow the seeds of healthy eating right from the womb. Do you know the baby can taste whatever you eat?"

Some women were flabbergasted. A few even looked at each other.

"Yes! Modern science has proven that the taste of amniotic fluid in which the baby floats changes according to the mother's diet[xxiv]. And baby gulps it all the time. The food you eat develops his taste preference and his preference for food will impact his choice of lifestyle."

"The taste buds can be cultivated," commented the Ancient Guru. "In India, we have different food in different regions. If we go to South India, we have idli, dosa, medu vada, rasam, etc. In North India, we have chole, paneer, samosa, etc. In West India, we have patra, khaman, locho, khandvi, dhokla, thepla, etc. So, when we travel, we can eat other regions' food for 10-15 days, but then we miss our native food because of the taste cultivated. It's the same for people across different nations. Everyone likes their traditional food more because of the taste cultivated in the womb. Baby develops his taste buds through his mother."

"So, my light warriors, the fourth ritual is to start eating consciously. Only eat what you want your baby to eat. If you want him to have soups, salads, green veggies, etc. start eating them right now. And if you want him to stay away from fried, high caloric food, chocolates, ice-creams, etc., then stop eating them right from today."

 RITUAL #4: Eat Consciously Every Time

The Ancient Guru paused for a moment. He saw some women making faces on avoiding chocolates and ice-creams. He inhaled deeply, **"Garbh Sanskar is never easy, but it's the right thing to do.** If you have that burning desire to give the best to the baby, if you want to make a difference, then this is what you need to do. So, will you eat consciously?" asked the Ancient Guru.

The crowd nodded.

The Ancient Guru explained, "Sattvic gunna represents balance. Eating more sattvic food brings a sense of balance and keeps you happy and calm. The sattvic food has the highest energy. They are fresh, simple, natural, contain little spices, and lightly cooked or raw foods. They contain more nutrients rich plant food and less processed food. They include fresh fruits and vegetables, salads, freshly cooked homemade food, honey, ghee, dates, turmeric, coriander, ginger, fennel, cardamom, green gram, pumpkin, wheat, etc.[xxv]"

"Rajasic gunna represents activity. Rajasic foods are spicy, hot, sour, bitter, and pungent. Rajasic foods are tea, coffee, pulses, onion, garlic, green chilies, black pepper, cocoa, soda, broccoli, cauliflower, spinach, pickles, chillies or anything else too spicy or hot. They bring movement to the body, help decision-making, perform daily tasks and facilitate mental robustness. You should eat rajasic food in moderation. When one eats more rajasic foods, one is prone to stress, anxiety, overwhelm and overexcitement."

"Tamas gunna is associated with laziness. They cause inertia in the body. Tamasic food has very low prana and acts as a sedative, inducing physical and mental sluggishness. They don't just include some food items; rather, anything eaten in excess turns tamasic. Tamasic foods are stale, packed, deep-fried, processed, etc. More tamasic food in one's diet causes laziness, weakness, stagnation, aging and pessimism."

Food Gunnas Table[xxvi]

Gunna	Association	Examples
Sattvic	Balance. It brings balance and calmness to the body	Fresh fruits and vegetables, salads, freshly cooked homemade food, honey, ghee, dates, turmeric, coriander, ginger, fennel, cardamom, green gram, pumpkin, wheat, etc.
Rajasic	Activity. It brings movement to the body.	Tea, coffee, pulses, onion, garlic, green chilies, black pepper, tobacco, cocoa, soda, broccoli, cauliflower, spinach, pickles, etc.
Tamasic	Laziness. It brings stability and repairs the body	Ice cream, chocolates, biscuits, chips, cheese, bread, samosas, kachoris, etc.

"How many of you have felt that when you eat deep-fried food in larger quantity, you feel sleepy?" asked the Ancient Guru.

Over 1500 women raised their hands.

"Exactly! That's the point here. Whenever you eat any high-calorie tamasic food such as ice-creams, cakes, or other desserts, you will feel lazy. Some examples of tamasic food are packed foods such as ice cream, chocolates, biscuits, chips, processed foods such as cheese and bread, and deep-fried foods such as samosas and kachoris. Whereas when you eat sattvic food, you will feel light on your stomach and high on energy. There is this age-old saying:"

'We Are What We Eat'

"Let me give you a scientific explanation. The food we eat is the grossest form. They turn into different energies and work as per their nature in a subtle form. Do you know the ghee we eat becomes our voice in a subtle form?[xxvii] Amazing, isn't it?"

It was an aha moment for the crowd. Earlier, most women thought it would be a dull session in which what they already knew would be repeated. But they were wrong. Whatever the Ancient Guru revealed had added a new perspective to their existing knowledge.

"Food you eat ultimately impacts the way you feel, the way you think, the way you behave and shapes the life you live. Here is the flow:"

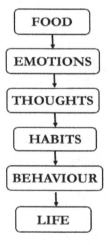

"We know that the food we eat plays a very crucial role yet, we consume unhealthy food frequently. **Eating right is a sign of respecting the body.** If you honor your body, start eating healthy from this very moment. However, don't just stick to sattvic food. Our diet must include all of the three categories of food. However, it would be best if you took care of the proportion. If you eat just sattvic food, you will stay happy and calm and neglect your work and responsibility. Rajasic food is essential for doing the work. In this world, we are to perform our roles. We must value our work and show up each day. If we don't eat tamasic food, we won't be able to sleep at night and suffer from insomnia. When consumed in moderation, tamasic food brings stability and helps the body repair itself. Thus, include all of them in your diet, watch the proportion, and modify accordingly."

A woman in a long white kurta asked, "Master, I understand the importance of good food, but I am just unable to do it. My craving for junk food isn't letting me eat healthily."

The Ancient Guru answered, "You suffer from cravings because of your past habits. Once you work on your habits, develop healthy rituals, and eat with mindfulness, you will win over your cravings. You won't crave it in the mornings or while at work. You will crave it mostly at night. The perfect solution is to sleep at that time and wake up early each day. You will be happier, healthier and proud of yourself. The nine months of your pregnancy are very crucial for the best development of the baby. So, during this phase, eat consciously and you will be fine."

"The food chart I have given is based on the energy of the food rather than nutrients. As per the Ayurvedic principles, we already know that our body can form anything it requires, provided it is healthy. Food in the chart is classified based on its prana value and vatta inducing properties. It's crucial to avoid food which causes gas."

"Why Master?" a woman in a black color jumpsuit from the second row asked.

"The nature of wind is to throw things away. The storm, the cyclone, etc., throw away everything on its way. Similarly, the gas in the body throws everything out and in the case of a very high vatta, it causes bleeding, premature delivery and in unfortunate circumstances, even miscarriages[xxviii]. Some women even face difficulty in conception due to high vatta."

The Ancient Guru closed his eyes for a moment feeling the pain of women who suffer miscarriages. "That is why the food chart focuses on the prana value and avoids vatta inducing food."

I. Vegetables

"Here is the Food Chart. Prepare your diet weekly using this chart for healthy and energetic pregnancy. The veggies have been divided into three categories. The first column includes those which you can eat in abundance without any restriction. The second column consists of those items you should eat in moderation. The third column consists of those you can just taste or avoid altogether."

"You should eat food which is local and seasonal. They are best for your body. Avoid eating imported food as your body isn't naturally accustomed to digest it. The climate, culture, and food habits of every region are different. Our body is habituated to the conditions where we live. That is why what's local and seasonal is the best food for our body."

"For vegetables, the chart gives so many options under the abundance section. So, you won't be out of choices at all. One recommendation is to add **curry leaves** wherever you can. They aid in digestion tremendously."

Abundance	Moderation	Restriction
Pumpkin	Cabbage	Okra (Bhindi)
Bottle Gourd (Dudhi)	Cauliflower	Flat Green Beans (Papdi)
Pointed Gourd (Parwar)	Potato	Green Cowpeas (Chodi)
Sponge Gourd	Tomato	Hyacinth Beans (Surati Papdi)
Ridge Gourd	Cucumber	Cluster Beans (Guvar)
Snake Gourd	Brinjal	Corn
Apple Gourd (Tinda)	Onion	Green Chickpeas
Spine Gourd (Kantola)	Garlic	Green Pigeon Peas (Tuvar)
Ash Gourd (Petha)	Radish	Peas
Ivy Gourd (Tindora)	Sweet Potato	Peanuts
Bitter Gourd (Karela)	Capsicum	
Drumstick (Sarogo)	Beetroot	
Broccoli	Carrot	
French Beans (Fansi)		
Leafy Vegetables		
Water Chestnut		
Jackfruit		
Fenugreek Leaves		
Gooseberry (Amla)		
Colocasia Leaves		
Cilantro		

Food mentioned here is just for reference purposes and is not a substitute for medical guidance.

"The enthusiastic mothers can grow '**Microgreens**' and add them to their diet. Microgreens are baby plants. When the seeds germinate and the plant develops its first true leaves, they are harvested because they are packed with concentrated nutrients and intense aroma. They are a 'super nutritious' superfood that contains zinc, potassium, antioxidants, and are 2-40 times more nutritious than the mature plant. This nutrient-packed bundle of leaves will easily fulfill all your nutritional requirements. It will also keep the fiber content high which in turn will ease your constipation and bloating issues[xxix]."

Grow Microgreens

1. Soak a handful of grains overnight.
2. Wash them well and spread them evenly on the tray.
3. Cover the grains with garden soil.
4. Spray water twice a day.
5. Keep the tray in partial sunlight.
6. The grains will start sprouting within a week.
7. You can harvest the leaves after the two first leaves mature.

Ananya asked, "Can you please tell us what we can eat during morning sickness?"

"Nice question! Whenever you feel discomfort and are not well, you can eat whatever you want. You can even eat your favorite food, which can be chinese, dosa, pani puri, etc. The only condition is that it must be homecooked. During the first trimester, most women face morning sickness. You can forget the chart entirely and eat whatever you feel like eating during that time. Just take care that it's home-cooked. Don't be too rigid because it won't benefit your baby. If you are in discomfort, you will transfer pain to the baby. We don't want that. The first rule of Garbh Sanskar is to be **HAPPY**. What you feel, your baby will also feel. So, you can eat to your heart's content when facing discomfort and gradually, when you feel healthy again, you can come back to the food chart."

II. Fruits

"You can eat all the local and seasonal fruits. However, some fruits must be taken in moderation because they are vatta inducing. No juices are allowed because it's tough for the body to digest juices and during pregnancy, you already have weak digestion. You must chew your fruits and veggies."

Vatta Inducing Fruits

1   Watermelon
2   Muskmelon
3   Pineapple
4   Papaya

"You can eat these fruits in the following quality:

Just two slices at a time and the size of the slice is a finger width."

The crowd laughed

Further, take care of the following:

1   Coconut water – You can have it before noon. The best time to have coconut water is one hour after sunrise. Please don't drink it on an empty stomach. And avoid it entirely if you have gastric issues.
2   Sugarcane[xxx] – Don't ever drink sugarcane juice because it's tough to digest due to its high sucrose content. You must always chew the sugarcane if you want to have it.
3   Mango – Avoid mango ras during pregnancy. You must soak the mango in water for an hour and then have it. It's best to limit the quantity to two mangoes in a day and eat only during its season.
4   Avoid fruits after 4 p.m. as they induce vatta.

5 No milkshakes, please! According to Ayurveda, fruits and milk are opposite in nature and shouldn't be mixed.

III. Flours

Flours that can be taken during pregnancy are:

Abundance	Moderation	Restriction
Whole Wheat Flour	Finger Millet Flour (Ragi)	All-purpose flour (Maida)
Rice Flour	Cornmeal Flour (Makki)	Corn Flour
Sorghum (Jowar) Flour	Bengal Gram Flour (Besan)	Cornstarch
	Pearl Millet Flour (Bajre)	
	Semonila Flour (Rawa)	
	Water Chestnut Flour	
	Amarnath Flour	

Avoid maida at all costs because it sticks to the microvilli in the intestines and causes indigestion.

IV. Rice

The local rice is best for digestion. There are several varieties of rice, with each region having its variety. Go out and look for local rice and you will have the best rice for your pregnancy. Just make sure you buy unpolished rice. Avoid basmati rice as it induces vatta. You can also have red and brown rice as they are rich sources of various nutrients but they are difficult to digest.

V.   Pulses

Pulses are one of the best sources of protein. But most of them increase vatta in the body. Because of this reason, they must be taken in moderation.

Abundance	Moderation	Restriction
Green Gram Whole (Moong)	Black Gram (Urad)	Soybeans
Green Gram Split (Chilka)	Bengal Gram (Chana)	Sprouts
Yellow Gram Split	Cowpeas (Choda)	
Horse Gram	Chickpeas (Chole)	
Pink Lentil (Masoor)	Hyacinth Beans (Val)	
Pigeon Peas Split (Tuvar dal)	White Peas (Vatana)	
	Bengal Gram Split	
	Tapioca Pearls (Sabudana)	

Moderation means having two teaspoons on your plate. You can fill your stomach with veggies and pulses under the abundance category. Also, those in moderation must be cooked in the following way to reduce their vatta properties:

Moderation Grain + Jeera + Hing + Garlic + Ginger + Ajwain

Your healthy gut means a healthy gut for the baby. You can avoid indigestion and constipation issues when you eat consciously. You can avoid those mentioned in the third column for at least nine months to keep your digestion healthy.

MIRACLE CONSTIPATION CURE[xxxi]
You can take one tablespoon of psyllium husk/isabgol with lukewarm milk at night in case of indigestion, bloating and constipation issues. The combination of milk and psyllium husk works like magic. If you are suffering from severe constipation, you can take it twice a day, once - the first thing in the morning and the second before going to bed.

VI. Dry fruits

You can eat dry fruits after soaking them overnight in the following quantities daily:

Quantity	Dryfruit
Number of your pregnancy month	Almonds
2-3	Cashew
1	Walnut
1	Fig
10-12	Black grapes
10-12	Monaka grapes

You can soak black grapes, monaka grapes and fig overnight and eat them in the morning after crushing them. They are perfect for digestion and ease constipation and bloating. You can also have one dry date. It's good to coat it with ghee. Do remember to avoid pistachio altogether.

In moderation, you can add various seeds such as watermelon, sunflower, pumpkin, flaxseed, etc.

VII. Liquids

A2 milk is best for consumption. Some other liquids you can have are buttermilk, lemon water, and fennel water. Add lots of ghee to your diet. Ghee aids in digestion and energizes your body.

Avoid tea and coffee entirely, or if that's not possible, limit them to half a cup in a day. The excessive consumption of tea and coffee hampers iron absorption and induces vatta in the body. But you all know that how you feel is most important throughout your pregnancy. If you follow the ideal diet and are unhappy, or your mind constantly goes to your morning tea/coffee, you do more harm than good. Do whatever you can with ease. Make efforts to bring some changes but don't expect everything to change overnight. Take baby steps, and you will reach there. Be happy and put conscious efforts for your best motherhood journey.

VIII.   Things to avoid

It's best if the following things are avoided:

1 Bakery products
2 Restaurant food
3 Stale food (when it has been more than 4 hours after the food is cooked, then it comes under this category)
4 Packed food (includes chocolates, ice-cream and chips)
5 Dairy products
6 Sweets cooked in shops
7 Fermented food
8 Bottled water (Research[xxxii] has proven its contamination with microplastics)

"Further, it is imperative to focus on how you eat. Don't watch any screen when you put anything into your stomach. Consider it this way; **eating is a sacred practice**. In ancient India, people used to eat food as medicine. They ate to live and today, most people live to eat. And what's the result? More lifestyle diseases such as diabetes, obesity, mental health issues, an aggressive world, more violence, high crime rates, etc. Can you see where we are going? And it all started with what we are eating, how we are eating, and our state of mind while eating," explained the Ancient Guru.

Some of the women started clapping.

The Ancient Guru grabbed this copper bottle and drank a few sips of water. "This is your homework for today. Make a sacred place for eating at your home and always eat at that place only. Don't eat on the bed or the couch. Also, avoid watching T.V, laptop, mobile phones, etc., while eating. It would be best if you didn't eat when sad or angry because it affects digestion. Chew 32 times. This will aid in digestion and your stomach will love you."

"Don't overeat. Further, don't drink water thirty minutes before and after eating. You can instead have 2-3 sips while eating. Become thankful for the food on your plate. And before eating, pray to the divine. More than one billion people on this planet aren't that lucky," said the Ancient Guru.

"There is a short food prayer called **Brahmaarpanam**[xxxiii]. We pray to Lord Brahma, the creator of this whole universe, through this prayer. You can learn it if you want your baby to know."

Brahmaarpanam Brahma Havir
Brahmaagnau Brahmanaa Hutam
Brahmaiva Tena Gantavyam
Brahma Karma Samaadhinaha
Aham Vaishvaanaro Bhutva
Praaninaam Dehamaashritha
Praanaapaana Samaa Yuktaha
Pachaamyannam Chatur Vidam
Harir Daatha Harir Bhoktha
Harir Annam Prajaapatih
Harir Vipra Shareerastu
Bhoonkte Bhojayathe Harih.

"If you find it too difficult, you can simply say '*Ann daata sukhi bhava*' before eating your meal. It means, may the one giving us food be happy."

"Praying will send a positive signal to the universe and invoke healthy emotions within you. Start eating consciously and food will start taking care of you. Start loving your body and your body will start loving you 10x. Whatever you give, you get it magnified. That's the law of nature. Today, lets' honor the food we eat," suggested the Ancient Guru.

"Sangachadwam."

The Ancient Guru joined his hands, blessed everyone and left the stage.

Ananya was tranquilized by the knowledge shared today. It hit her hard. Today's session was a complete eye-opener for her. She used to eat very quickly sometimes she ate while standing or driving because of work pressure. She drank water while standing most of the time after her meals. And when she had time, she used to watch her screen. She thought she was multitasking and making the most of her time. Now, she knew how wrong she was. These habits might have played a role in her struggle to conceive despite her every report being normal.

She always used to ask what was wrong with her. What was she doing wrong? But she had no answers. Now she did. She felt blessed. She promised to respect food, pray before eating, and have no screen time at the dining table.

DO IT RIGHT

1. We eat food for energy. Ayurveda divides food into three categories - Sattvic, Rajasic and Tamasic food.
2. One should have the highest proportion of sattvic food with some rajasic food and very little tamasic food in one's diet.
3. Eating right is a sign of respecting the body.
4. The nature of the vatta is to throw everything out and in the case of a very high vatta, it can cause bleeding, premature delivery and in unfortunate circumstances, even miscarriages.
5. You should eat food that is local and seasonal.
6. Add curry leaves and microgreens to your diet wherever you can.
7. The first rule of Garbh Sanskar is to be happy.
8. Make a sacred place for eating at your home and always eat at that place only.
9. Avoid watching the TV, laptop, mobile phones, etc., while eating. It would be best if you didn't eat when sad or angry because it affects digestion. Always chew 32 times.
10. Before eating, pray to the divine. Become thankful for the food on your plate.

CHAPTER 6

CHAKRAS HEALING

Today, the Ancient Guru had asked them to bring a woolen mat, Riya wondered why. She was reading a comic book. *We might attain another breakthrough and let go of our limitations.* Riya could already feel a tremendous difference between her earlier self and her present self. She was much liberated Riya. She regretted missing this workshop during her first pregnancy but was happy to attend it this time. Her conflicts with Varun had also decreased and she remained content most of the time. Her gynecologist also told her that the baby was developing very well and there was nothing to worry about.

"Good morning, darling!" Varun kissed her on her forehead breaking her train of thought. Riya hugged him and got ready for today's session with a woolen mat.

The Ancient Guru wore a white kurta pyjama today. Everyone felt a tremendous gush of uplifting energy in his presence. He was sitting in sukhasana on a big round woolen mat with a mandala knitted on it. It was about eight feet in diameter.

The volunteers gave the light warriors a picture as they entered the park and asked the crowd to settle down on the woolen mat, close their eyes for a few minutes, and focus on their breath. It had a human outline and seven different colored circles at various locations.

Ananya was enjoying the cool breeze touching her softly. She was completely engrossed in nature. She was listening to the melodious chirping of birds, losing herself in the aromatic freshness of morning dew. The strands of her hair were playing with her right cheek. And she heard the soothing sound of the Ancient Guru.

"Good morning, my light warriors! Gently you all may open your eyes," greeted the Ancient Guru.

"We all know a lot about our physical body. I am sure your gynecologist must also have briefed you enough about your physical body. But we hardly think of our other bodies!" exclaimed the Ancient Guru.

The crowd looked at each other in confusion. Ananya wondered whether she heard it right. "Other bodies?"

"Yes! Our existence is not limited to just this physical form. There are three different types of bodies. The first type is the gross or physical body, which we all know. The second type is the subtle body that gives energy to our gross body and the third type is the causal body where our soul resides[xxxiv]."

Riya said, "Master, I couldn't understand."

The Ancient Guru explained, "We are not open to new knowledge at many times. And that is why we find it hard to comprehend. This knowledge is profound. Let me explain with an analogy. Suppose that you are using your laptop; the laptop is the physical form. Still, it requires the software and electricity to work, right? Its software is a subtle form. But there is something else also. Who is operating it? It's you and that is the causal body. Are you getting it now?"

"Wow!" exclaimed a few women from the fourth row. Most of them were so amazed that they couldn't react at all. They didn't move an inch and were all ears.

"We all know a lot about the physical body so let's look at the subtle body today. It comprises of over **72,000 nadis** or the energy channels, **seven major chakras** and **prana energy** or the life force. The prana flows throughout the body and the chakras through these nadis. Everything on this planet, whether living or non-living, has prana. When we learn how to tap into the abundance of prana of the universe, we will always remain full of vigor."

The Ancient Guru paused and made eye contact with every participant. He loved sharing this part of knowledge the most because he thought it was the single most essential piece of knowledge that everyone on this planet should know. This knowledge, when applied daily, changes the life of the person who practices it completely. Through this knowledge, one can heal oneself and others also.

"Chakra is a vortex of energy. Do you all know how electricity is transmitted? Electricity isn't transmitted to your house directly from the point of its generation. It first goes to the power stations and then is transmitted through the transmission lines to your home. Similarly, the prana energy from the universe enters the body through chakras, which act as a power station that further distributes the prana to different parts of the body through nadis. There are seven chakras in the physical body located at seven different places[xxxv]. Let's look at them in-depth."

"You can imagine these chakras to be located in one line on the spinal cord for better imagination. You can have a look at the picture for a better understanding. Each chakra has different characteristics like color, petals, shape, elements, etc. Today we will understand its location and the emotions associated with them. It will help you get over your emotions and live a happier and more fulfilling life."

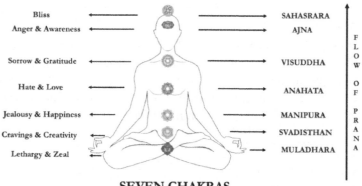

SEVEN CHAKRAS

The Ancient Guru paused for a moment. He let the crowd absorb what he revealed. He picked up his copper bottle and gulped some water soothing his dry throat. He kept it aside and said, "Do you want some examples of the emotional connection with chakras?"

"Yes!" shouted the crowd of over 1500 women.

"But before that, let me tell you one special thing about Sahasrara chakra. It has just one positive emotion - bliss. It has no negative emotion. But even the Manipura chakra has happiness linked with it. Can you tell what is the difference between the bliss at Sahasrara and happiness at Manipura Chakra? Any guesses?"

Most of them were clueless. Everyone wanted to know more. All adult women grasped this highest knowledge with the utmost attention just like children.
"No idea? Alright! The happiness associated with Manipura chakra is dependent on the people, things and circumstances. In contrast, the happiness/bliss associated with the Sahasrara chakra is beyond these three elements. It is the eternal joy from which no one wants to escape. Everyone desires that kind of blissful state of mind. However, beware: this state of mind isn't achieved by running after it. It is achieved through **consistent practice and conscious decisions.**"

The crowd was mesmerized by this new revelation. Riya started whistling again. Ananya wasn't offended this time. She smiled at this gesture of Riya. She even requested Riya to teach her how to whistle.

"Now let's see some of the relatable examples on emotions and chakras. Did anyone of you feel that your throat was choked up when you were extremely sad?"

Around 1500 women raised their hands.

"Yes! Do you ever have the same feeling when you were truly grateful for something?"

This time around 1000 women raised their hands.

"Now, can you see the connection? When you strongly feel those emotions, you will feel the sensation in the region of their location. There is little pain in the heart region when you hate someone so much. Similarly, when you are jealous of someone, you can feel a pit in your stomach. So, my light warriors, start observing your emotions and you will be able to see the connection every time."

It was an AHA moment for every woman who came today for the session.

Ananya raised her right hand and asked, "Master, this knowledge is amazing. Can you please teach us how we can turn a negative emotion into positive emotion?"

"Excellent question!" the Ancient Guru exclaimed. "Emotions are like flowing rivers. They cannot be stopped, just like we cannot stop the river's flow. But they can be directed by simple awareness. You can change the way you respond by becoming aware of your emotions. When you know about your emotions, your energy is channelized to the positive side of the Ajna chakra. Through this knowledge, you will stop reacting and start responding. We will practice it at the end of the session."

"Let's first look at the flow of prana. The prana raises upward on the positive side of the emotions and goes down on the negative side of the feelings."

Ex. If you are happy, your heart fills with love and then you will be grateful to the divine.

Ex2. When you are filled with anger, if you don't become aware, you will suddenly feel the hurt and might start crying, and then the hatred comes in, which, if not tackled, can turn into more negative emotions.

"I am sure most of you have experienced this. The only difference was at that time, you were not aware of it and didn't know how to deal with it, but now you know."

"So, the fifth ritual is healing your chakras. Before we start our practice, you can quickly take a short break," directed the Ancient Guru.

 RITUAL #5: Heal Your Chakras

Some women started munching fruits and dry fruits. And some went near the waterfall to enjoy nature. A few went to use the restroom.

After ten minutes, everyone settled on their woolen mats and the Ancient Guru was back on the stage.

"Isn't anyone curious to know why woolen mats? If anyone wants to know, raise your hand straight towards the sky," directed the Ancient Guru.

Around 900 women raised their hands.

"Well, not everyone wants to know," chuckled the Anci. Guru.

The remaining women also raised their hands.

"Okay, relax! We all know that wool is an excellent insulator. Do you all remember that earth is an excellent conductor of electricity? We all had learned this in the fifth or sixth standard. We use the woolen mat to conserve the energy tapped from the universe into our body and stop it from flowing into the earth."

There was another AHA moment for the crowd.

"Always do your practice on the woolen mat. It will fill your body with prana and give you the results of your practice."

The Ancient Guru instructed everyone to relax completely and take their attention inwards.

CHAKRA HEALING PRACTICE

Let's sit easily and comfortably in sukhasana. Those who cannot sit on the mat can use the chair. Keep your spine straight and body relaxed. Keep your palms on your knees facing the sky. Take a few long deep breaths. Become aware of your breath, your thoughts, your emotions. Keep breathing. Relax your eyes, forehead, your shoulders. Now gently take your attention to the Muladhara chakra. Take a few deep breaths there, move to Svadisthan chakra, and take a few breaths. Gradually bring your attention to all the chakras, one by one. After completing, you may lay down on your mat and relax completely for 5-10minutes.

Ananya had a profound experience. She had never felt something like this before. It all seemed magical to her. After she opened her eyes, she found the whole world to be a new place. She looked at the infinity tattoo on her right wrist. *Finally, this symbol got its meaning.* She found infinity within her finite life.

The Ancient Guru asked, "How is everyone feeling?"

Everyone did a thumbs up.

"Your sparkling faces say it all," expressed the Ancient Guru. "Do remember this experience and practice chakras healing for at least ten minutes daily. It will heal your body, your emotions, and your soul. It is very beneficial for you and your baby. Just doing it once in a while makes no difference. It takes consistency and determination to bring a difference in one's life. So please don't stop here. Go ahead and win over your limitations and become limitless. Become a Supermom!"

"Sangachadwam."

The Ancient Guru blessed everyone and left.

DO IT RIGHT

1. There exist three different types of bodies – physical, subtle and causal body.

2. The subtle body comprises 72,000 nadis or the energy channels, seven major chakras and prana energy or the life force.

3. The chakras are the vortex of energy.

4. The prana energy from the universe enters the body through chakras, which act as a power station that further distributes the prana to different parts of the body through nadis.

5. Emotions are like a flowing river. They cannot be stopped but they can be directed by simple awareness.

6. Always use the woolen mat to conserve the energy tapped from the universe into our bodies while meditating.

CHAPTER 7
POWER OF BREATH

Arjun was enjoying the positive change in Ananya. Seeing her happy filled his heart with joy. He hated when she used to crib over petty things and wasted her precious energy. He expressed gratitude to the divine and planned to take Ananya out for a romantic dinner on the beach. Ananya was very excited about the surprise. She wore a long black fish-cut gown, carried a silver clutch, and put on light makeup. When Arjun picked Ananya up from her office, she loved the way he smelled. Arjun still used the same musk perfume which she had gifted him two years back. Arjun wore a black shirt and dark blue jeans to twin with Ananya.

Ananya didn't know about the location yet. *Where would have Arjun planned the dinner?* Arjun drove the car to La Emerald Hotel. It was located on the beach and offered private bedding on the sand under the sky. There was an elegant table for two with floral table décor and candles. Beside the table was cozy bedding decorated with a white net and fairy lights. As soon as she saw the romantic setup, her eyes lit up. She was amazed by the details of the surprise.

Arjun went towards the table and pulled the chair for Ananya. She blushed and settled down. After dinner, Arjun asked her for a dance. *I feel like a princess.* She gently held his hand and moved her feet on the cold sand. A romantic Greek song was playing in the background and they both danced under the moonlight. She found the dance, the music, the sand, the ocean and Arjun, very therapeutic.

Later they settled on the bed. The beach was pitch black and only white streaks of the waves were visible due to phosphorescence and the moonlight. There was no sound other than those of waves.

Ananya rested her head on Arjun's chest and said, "I am awestruck by this surprise. Thank you so much, Arjun, for making it so special."

"Anything for you, love. You are putting so much effort for the baby's best development. Can't I put some effort to shower my love upon you?" *I love that smile on your face Ananya. It gives me immense joy.*

Ananya's cheeks turned crimson, just like a sixteen-year-old teenager.

"I am proud of you, Ananya. It's not easy to make such lifestyle changes. But you did it for our baby. I love you to the moon and back."

"Thanks, Arjun. Look at the gazillion stars above."

Arjun turned his gaze from Ananya to the sky. There were no clouds and millions of stars were visible in the sky.

"They look like a painting!" exclaimed Arjun.

Ananya kissed him on her cheeks and whispered, "You are awesome."

Arjun smiled and suggested, "Now we should sleep because you have a session at 5 a.m."

Ananya nodded. Arjun kissed her on her forehead and wrapped his arms around her womb. He cuddled Ananya and the love birds slept under the sky.

Next morning

The Ancient Guru was back to his maroon kasaya attire today. Riya noticed that the woolen mats were still there. *We might learn something related to energy again.* She was very excited to learn more. *I feel blessed for being here in these mastery sessions for my baby's best development. I didn't know a mother could have such an impact on the fetus. I feel powerful and important. I can impact the whole world through my motherhood. I feel as if my life has been given a new meaning.*

"Good Morning, my light warriors!" greeted the Ancient Guru. "I hope you all are following what we have learned till now."

"Yes!" said the crowd cheerfully.

Ananya reached for the session directly from the hotel. She managed to arrive just on time. She searched for Riya and sat beside her, a little distracted; still thinking about the last night.

"Today, we will learn another essential aspect connected with energy but more focused on the breath. We all know that breath gives us energy. Physiologically, it fills our lungs with oxygen-rich air and takes carbon dioxide-rich air out of the body. The oxygen collected in the alveoli is distributed through blood capillaries to the other body parts. Do you all agree?"

The Ancient Guru looked at everyone. He could see the nods of many women.

"But have you ever connected your breath with your emotions? Have you ever noticed that when you are angry, your breath becomes fast and shallow, or when you are scared, it almost stops?"

A few women in the third row laughed.

"Or when you are doing what you love, when you are relaxed, it is very deep and soothing? Isn't it amazing? Do you know we can change how we feel by changing how we breathe?" asked the Ancient Guru.

Many women become attentive. A few were skeptical.

"Yes! It's truly powerful. Try this when you are angry next time – pause for a moment, become aware of your shallow breathing and consciously take a few long deep breaths and you will significantly calm yourself down. Similarly, when you are upset about something, focus on your breathing and you will be just fine. You are powerful. **All the power you need is already within you.**"

Ananya thought *I might be able to manage stress more effectively by focusing on my breath. I will follow this consciously whenever I get angry, I promise.* She was wearing a yellow jumpsuit with a golden and cream color belt.

"We all have heard about the term pranayama. But do we know what it exactly means? The word prana can be divided into two parts – Prana and Yama. Prana means the life force, and Yama means control. It's popularly known as **controlled breathing**. Through pranayama, we can manage our emotions, thoughts and well-being better. But, there is another beautiful meaning. The term can also be broken into **Prana** and **Ayama**. Prana means life force and Ayama implies dimension, so it means moving in the **dimension of the life force**. Amazing right?"

A few women said, "WOW."

Such a definition was interesting, Ananya said to herself.

"Now, we will be learning one very important pranayama for the best development of the mother and the baby. Many of the pranayamas cannot be done during pregnancy. But this is the

109

safest and most effective pranayama, if you do it every day for the next nine months, your baby will do it with you when he turns two. Who doesn't want their baby to do pranayamas? Please raise your hands."

No one raised their hands.

"No one right? We all want our babies to do pranayama because it helps us in many ways."

The Ancient Guru said, "Today, we are going to learn **Anulom Vilom pranayama**[xxxvi]. It is known as balancing pranayama because it balances both sides of our brain. Some of its other benefits are[xxxvii]:

i.   Relaxes the body completely
ii. Calms the body
iii. Improves sleep quality
iv. Increases the lung capacity, which is very important for the pregnancy as in later stages breathing becomes difficult due to expanding uterus.
v.   Eases labor pain
vi. Adds to skin glow
vii. Heals the body
viii. Relieves migraine
ix. Relieves stress
x.   Maintains blood pressure
xi. Optimizes functioning of cardiovascular systems
xii. Promotes overall well-being"

PRACTICE TIME

Let's sit comfortably on our woolen mats in sukhasana. Keep the left hand on the left knee facing the sky. Take the first two fingers of the right hand and place them between the eyebrows, thumb on the right nostril and ring finger on the left nostril. Inhale and exhale. Inhale from the left nostril and exhale from the right. Now inhale from the right nostril and exhale from the left. This makes one round of Anulom Vilom pranayama. Repeat it for nine rounds in your rhythm. Keep your breath deep and slow. After completing the rounds, you may relax your hands and feel the sensations in your body.

Riya was finding it hard to breathe deeply. So, many thoughts were running in her mind. One of the volunteers came close to her, and she took deep breaths close to her ears. Riya followed the rhythm and could do it better now.

The volunteer whispered, "Don't worry! You will get better at it with practice," and Riya smiled.

There was complete silence. The only sound audible was of the waterfall and the chirping of birds. The park was energized by the motivated mothers who were willing to do whatever it took for the best development of their babies and serve society. It felt as if the universe was watching them and the angels were supporting them in their endeavor.

After ten minutes, the Ancient Guru made mothers aware of their surroundings and asked them to open their eyes gently. He asked, "How was everyone feeling? This is your sixth ritual."

 RITUAL #6: Practice Nine Rounds Of Anulom Vilom Pranayama Daily

111

One woman in a long suit in the fifth row said, "It's so relaxing! I haven't been this relaxed in a long time. Thank you so much for this wonderful experience, Master."

Another woman from the first row raised her hand. The Ancient Guru made eye contact with her and nodded at her to speak.

The woman said, "You are an amazing mentor! This pranayama has such a tranquilizing effect. I didn't wish to come out of that state of mind."

The Ancient Guru smiled, "That's great! Do add it to your daily routine. If you want to know more, raise your hands."

The crowd raised their hands almost instantly.

The Ancient Guru was happy to create curiosity amongst the young mothers. *Their lives would never be the same again and this world will become a better place to live in.*

"Do you know about gestures?" asked the Ancient Guru.

One lady wearing a purple saree said, "They are hand movements like handshakes."

The Ancient Guru said, "Absolutely correct! Let's learn about '**Mudras.**' Mudras are hand gestures used to channel the prana energy from the universe to a specific part of the body[xxxviii]. They keep the body in the receptive mode so that body is ready to tap into the abundant energy of the universe. There are more than 1000 mudras in our ancient scriptures. Today, we will learn six of them which are most useful in pregnancy."

"Are you all ready?" asked the Ancient Guru.

"Yes!" the crowd of women roared in unison.

1   Gyan Mudra

The first mudra that we are going to learn is the **Gyan mudra**. It is known as the mudra of knowledge. It improves concentration and sharpens memory.

GYAN MUDRA

> **Hand Position**
> Take your first finger, join it with the thumb and place your palms on your knees.

The Ancient Guru touched his right hand's first finger and thumb and showed it to the crowd. He said, "This is the Gyan mudra. Could you show me the mudra, everyone?"

The volunteers keenly observed everyone and corrected the incorrect gestures. We will take ten long deep breaths in each mudra, but we will learn about all the mudras before starting our practice.

Benefits:

  i.   Improves concentration
  ii.   Stimulates the pituitary gland
  iii. Relieves tension and depression
  iv.   Boosts immunity
  v.   Relives mental disorders
  vi.   Cures heart diseases
  vii. Prepares the body for meditation

2   Prana Mudra

The Prana mudra increases the prana energy in the body.

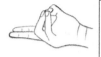

PRANA MUDRA

Hand Position
Place your first two fingers straight and curl the last two fingers touching the thumb.

Benefits:

i. Increases prana in every cell of the body.
ii. Heals the body
iii. Reduces eyesight issues
iv. Enhances blood flow
v. Boosts immunity
vi. Improves awareness, focus and productivity
vii. It brings more stability and balance to the mind
viii. Cures sleep disorders
ix. Strengthens the body
x. Removes blockages in the energy channels
xi. Removes fatigue
xii. Eases muscles pain

"Whenever you feel low on energy, just remember this mudra for you. Once you know how it's done, you can instantly tap into the abundant universal energies through this mudra," suggested the Ancient Guru.

3   Chinmay mudra

The Chinmay mudra enhances the awareness in the body and the mind. It creates a sense of balance and alignment in the body.

CHINMAY MUDRA

Hand Position
Touch your first finger and thumb and curl the rest of the three fingers inwards.

Benefits:

i.   Enhances awareness
ii.   Calms the mind
iii. Relieves stress and anxiety
iv.   Increases prana
v.   Enhances lung capacity
vi.   Stimulates thoracic region and optimizes its functioning
vii. Boosts metabolism
viii. Facilitates optimal functioning of the nervous system
ix.   Cures insomnia
x.   Cures anger issues

4 Adi mudra

The Adi mudra channelizes the prana in the mind region. It is often called the **first mudra** because the fetus can make this hand gesture right in the womb. You can sit in Adi mudra and take a few deep breaths whenever you have any headaches. Your headache will lessen in intensity, and it will cure completely over a period of regular practice.

ADI MUDRA

| **Hand Position** |
| Put your thumb at the beginning of your last finger and roll your fingers towards the palm. |

Benefits:

i.   It calms the mind
ii.   Prepares the body for profound meditations
iii. Enhances oxygen flow in the body
iv.   Increases mental awareness
v.   Balances both the hemispheres of the brain
vi.   Rejuvenates the nervous system

115

vii. Increases the lungs' capacity
viii. Optimizes the functioning of vital organs
ix. Energizes the Sahasrara chakra

5 Merudanda Mudra

The Merudanda mudra is also called **spine mudra**. It heals and strengthens the spine.

MERUDANDA MUDRA

Hand Position
We all know how to give a thumbs up, right? Thumbs up gesture of the hand is Merudanda mudra.

Benefits:

i. It strengthens the spine
ii. Cures back pain
iii. Improves bone health.
iv. Improves focus and concentration
v. Activates all the chakras
vi. Relieves slip disc issues
vii. Aids in detoxification of the body
viii. Improves the functioning of circulatory and respiratory systems
ix. Reduces obesity
x. It has a soothing effect on the nervous system

6 Apana Mudra

The Apana mudra facilitates the free flow of Apana vayu. It is also called a cleansing or purification gesture. It also aids in the childbirth process.

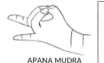
APANA MUDRA

| **Hand Position** |
| Take your second and third fingers and touch them with your thumb. |

We will not practice this mudra. Women in the mid of their 8th month of pregnancy can start this mudra practice daily for ten minutes.

Benefits:

i. This mudra helps in the normal delivery of the baby.
ii. Optimizes the functioning of the small and large intestines
iii. Relives constipation
iv. Relives indigestion and acidity
v. Regulates menstrual cycle in women
vi. Strengthens pelvic organs
vii. Relieves back pain
viii. Strengthens the immune system
ix. Cleanses the body and aids in the removal of toxins
x. Releases emotional blockages

"Apana vayu is part of our subtle body. It is responsible for the expulsion of wastes such as urine, stool, sweat and menstrual blood in women and sperm in men. It also helps in the expulsion of the fetus from the uterus at the time of childbirth. Apana mudra shall be practiced only from the **mid of the 8th month of pregnancy**. It is so powerful that if practiced earlier the baby can born pre-mature. Practicing this mudra activates the Apana vayu in the body and facilitates the normal delivery of the baby."

Ananya noted not to practice this mudra earlier in bold on her phone and asked Riya to remind her and be cautious.

The Ancient Guru took a breath and said, "These were some of the most important mudras which you must practice during pregnancy. This is your seventh ritual."

 ## RITUAL #7: Practice Mudra Pranayama Daily

"Further, when you place the palms open on the knees, that's called **Maha mudra** practiced to tap abundance energy from the universe into our body.We learned about the Chin mudra, Chinmay mudra, Prana mudra, Adi mudra, Merudanda mudra and Apana mudra. Now let's practice them. We will practice the first five mudras and avoid Apana mudra practice," said the Ancient Guru.

Ananya was recalling the mudras.

Riya asked, "Do you think they will work?"

Riya believed the Ancient Guru on most things, but it was difficult for her to trust the effectiveness of the mudras.

"I trust my Master completely, Riya," said Ananya. "Even though my logical mind might be unable to accept certain things, I will still follow him because he has made me experience things which I have never felt before in my life. Also, we don't understand much about the subtle body and the energy channels, but they do exist. We all have experienced it."

"You are right," affirmed Riya. "I should stop doubting the mudras and don't let my faith waver. Thank you, Ananya, for guiding me."

"Always," grinned Ananya.

MUDRA PRACTICE

Let's sit easily and comfortably in sukhasana. Place both the palms on the knee facing the sky, spine erect and shoulders relaxed. Gently you may close your eyes and take a few long deep breaths. Now place your hands in Gyan mudra. If you don't remember, you can open your eyes to see the mudra and continue the practice. Take ten long deep breaths. Now keep your hands in Prana mudra. Inhale and exhale completely. Continue breathing in your rhythm. Now place your hands in Chinmay mudra. Take ten deep breaths. Now place your hands in Adi mudra and take ten deep breaths. Now make Merudanda mudra and continue taking long deep breaths.

There was quiescence in the park. It was as if the divine witnessed these dedicated mothers and showered his blessings. Nature was playing the sound of love. Soft, soothing winds, chirping birds, the sound of the waterfall and the rays of the sun all were dancing in joy and kissing the souls of these new young mothers who wanted the best for their babies. Garbh Sanskar is not easy to practice. It's not easy to wake up early in the morning and come for the session. It's not easy to blindly trust the Master and surrender completely. It's not easy to be consistent with rituals. It's not easy to learn new things. It's not easy to dive into the unknown. None of these is easy, yet they all are here because they have experienced it and have felt that being here is a blessing. By following the Ancient Guru, they can give the best to their children. They want to serve society. They want to impact the lives of millions through their motherhood. They want to be a proud mother. So that when they see their baby revolutionizing the world, they can pat themselves and say that they did their job well. They chose Garbh Sanskar over gossip. They chose Garbh Sanskar over watching TV. They chose Garbh Sanskar over social media. **Garbh Sanskar is not easy, but it's the right thing to do**. They are genuinely the supermoms!

119

After fifteen minutes, the Ancient Guru made everyone aware of their bodies and their surroundings and instructed women to gently open their eyes with a big smile on their faces.

"How is everyone? Are you feeling better? I could see the radiance on your faces. Your smile says it all," said the Ancient Guru.

All the women were completely relaxed. They felt light from within.

"How can we experience this, Master! It's so unbelievable," asked Riya.
The Ancient Guru smiled and said, "Mudras tap into the abundant energy of the universe and channel the prana in specific regions of the body. When we surrender ourselves completely, we allow this prana to flow freely throughout our bodies. It removes all the toxins accumulated and reinvigorates the gross body. It will be very helpful if you add mudra practice to your daily routine. You will feel peaceful and relaxed. Mudra practice will facilitate the healthy development of the baby and bring more positivity in your life."

"Sangachadwam."

The Ancient Guru joined his hands in Namaste mudra and left the stage.

Riya asked, "Ananya, can we practice pranayamas and mudras together? It will be fun and we can be consistent too."

"Sure! At what time shall we practice?" asked Ananya.

"Evening works for me," answered Riya.

Ananya took a deep breath and exhaled completely. "I think it will be better if we can practice at this time since we have these

120

sessions only for the next two days. So, this time would be wonderful to practice."

Riya said, "Oh! I just forgot that these sessions were going to end."

"That's true! These sessions are amazing. We will miss them a lot," said Ananya

"Yeah! We will practice at this time. Let's meet in the garden or any other natural environment," suggested Riya.

"If you are comfortable, we can practice in my penthouse. The terrace has beautiful sunrise and sunset and the ocean view is just breathtaking," said Ananya

She asked Ananya where does she stay and it turned out that they stayed just one building away. Riya hugged Ananya and said she was very excited to practice together.

"Wow!! That would be great," Riya raised her hands for a high five.

Ananya gave a high five and they left the park.

DO IT RIGHT

1. Our breath and emotions are connected. We can change the way we feel by changing our breathing patterns.
2. You are powerful. All the power you need is already within you.
3. Prana means the life force, and Yama means control. It's popularly known as controlled breathing. It also means moving in the dimension of the life force.
4. Anulom Vilom pranayama is balancing pranayama because it balances both sides of our brain.
5. Mudras are hand gestures used to channel the prana energy from the universe to a specific part of the body.
6. Important mudras are Gyan, Prana, Chinmay, Adi and Merudanda mudra
7. Apana vayu is responsible for the expulsion of wastes such as urine, stool, sweat and menstrual blood in women and sperm in men. It helps remove the fetus from the uterus at the time of childbirth.
8. Apana mudra regulates Apana vayu and shall be practiced only from the mid of the 8th month of pregnancy

Chapter 8
PREGNANCY DINCHARYA

Ananya was watching the sunset from her terrace. She loved spending time with nature. Sunsets took all her work stress away. She was curious to know more about the Ancient Guru. *Why he wore simple clothes and how he had amassed so much knowledge about Garbh Sanskar. I would go for the session early and ask the volunteers.* Arjun came from his office and hugged Ananya from behind, breaking her train of thought. They both dined together and played chess. They used to love the game of chess. Even when they were dating, they had made it a point to play chess every week. Their tradition of weekly chess continued after marriage. Sometimes they added music in the background and had chips while playing chess. But today, their tummies were already full, so it was just light saxophone music playing in the background. Ananya won the first game.

Arjun said, "This time, I will surely win."

Ananya chuckled.

The second game didn't have any winners and it was a draw. Then they had a romantic dance on their terrace under the moonlight. The moon was making Ananya's face glow. The fairy lights on the terrace were blinking with joy. She loved the smell of the ocean. She was dancing gently and was lost in the melody of the music. Love was in the air. Later, they both went to sleep in their cozy bed.

The following day, Ananya woke up early to satisfy her curiosity about the Ancient Guru. As planned, Ananya reached the park before time. She was wearing a naturally dyed muslin shirt and brown chinos. She searched for volunteers and asked three of them but they didn't know much. An old lady was observing Ananya. She waved at Ananya and signaled her to come to her. Ananya looked at her and nodded. She had never seen that old lady before in the sessions. She walked carefully, thinking whether the lady knew about the Ancient Guru.

The old lady with white hair and a wrinkled face wore a khadi saree. She was just like any next-door granny. She asked Ananya to take a seat beside her.

"Good Morning, young lady! What are you looking for?" asked the old lady warmly.

Ananya answered, "Good Morning! I wanted to know more about the Ancient Guru. How has he attained this mastery? Where is his family? What is his purpose?"

"Oh! so many questions are running in your head, my dear," exclaimed the old lady.

"Why do you want to know all this?" she inquired.

"I want to know so that I can tell my baby about him. I want my baby to know him. Also, I am curious and I am losing sleep over it," said Ananya making a face of discontent by moving her lips towards her chin.

The old lady laughed at her innocence and said, "Okay! I will answer your questions but don't make it a topic of gossip. Do you promise?"

"Yes, of course," promised Ananya.

"Meet me tomorrow after your session ends at this very place," said the old lady.

Ananya thanked the old lady and joined the others for the session.

The Ancient Guru was on the stage and most of the women had already taken their seats but Riya had reserved a spot for Ananya. On looking at her, Riya waved and Ananya settled.

"Why are you so late today?" asked Riya.

There was a pause.

Ananya thought for a moment and replied, "Just the morning sickness." *I didn't wish to lie but I had promised the old lady.*

Riya rubbed Ananya's back and they both looked towards the Ancient Guru.

"Good morning, my light warriors! I hope you are enjoying our mastery sessions so that you can serve this world and add more value to your life. Today, we will look into dincharya which one must follow during pregnancy. Pregnancy can be challenging at times. Struggles for small things, physical changes, emotional bursts and health issues are real. It's not easy to raise a baby within you. But with powerful rituals, you can overcome challenges with a smile on your face and love in your heart. You won't be irritated, cranky, sad, or overwhelmed if you follow whatever you learn here and practice it diligently. You know, if you are unhappy, it affects the baby negatively."

The Ancient Guru paused for a moment and made an eye contact with all the women present in the session.

"On the other hand, if the mother is calm and composed, full of energy, faces challenges with a smile, the baby will be full of love. He will be a warrior just like you but better, smatter and stronger than you," the Ancient Guru raised both hands and spread them from inside out, covering the entire crowd.

The whole environment and the women were all ears. Few butterflies came near the Master and sat on his right hand. He grinned.

"Most women during pregnancy spend their time watching screens, mindlessly eating junk food, engaging in gossip and emotional drama. This is one of the core reasons why the world is the way it is right now. Lifestyle changes have affected everyone severely. As a result, there has been a proliferation of restaurants and hospitals. Do you see the nexus here?"

The crowd gasped.

"First, you spend your hard-earned money on food by going to restaurants or through food delivery apps. The food you consume is of tamasic gunna with low nutrients and is the root cause of diseases. You contract diseases because of your lifestyle. Later, you spend your money and time in the hospital to treat your body. All of this happened because we could not control our minds over our cravings. We were not aware and we gave in to your senses. Are you getting the point here?"

"Yes," a few women said. Many more nodded.

"Yes! and yet we keep doing that to ourselves. That is why we will look into what queens used to do to give birth to the baby with the qualities of a king. Today, we all know that our brain is divided into the right and the left hemispheres. The right hemisphere governs creativity and the left side governs logic and decision making. In a layman's language, the balance between them is crucial. Usually, we see that those involved in creative work, such as musicians, artists, etc., are weak at math and logical thinking. Similarly, those involved in analytical work like chartered accounts and lawyers have a powerful rational mind but suffer in creativity."

The Ancient Guru went to the stage's right corner, brought a small balancing machine, and showed it to the crowd. He placed the brain model on both sides and the machine was in perfect balance. He said, "Look here, they are in perfect harmony. If you achieve this, your Sushumna nadi[xxxix] will be activated and you will have access to the abundant energy of the universe 24*7. But please don't run after perfection. Just practice consistently and the universe will shower blessings on you and do wonders in the baby's brain development."

"So, the foremost thing to add in your pregnancy dincharya is to spend time with nature," declared the Ancient Guru.

 RITUAL #8: Spend Time With Nature Daily

"**Nature is the mother of creativity,** just like necessity is the mother of invention. Feel the breeze, watch nature closely. Walk barefoot on the grass; smell the first dewdrops of the day; get drenched in the rain; go star gazing and search for constellations; become sun-kissed; dive in the sea; sing with birds and dance with nature. Let nature become the witness of your bravery, commitment, unconditional joy, motherhood, and intense desire to serve society. It will brew more creativity within you, give you inner happiness and make you stronger. If you feel like you can even spend time with animals. Fall in love with their innocence and loyalty."

"You will find your soul blossoming from within when you are soaked in nature. This world will never be the same for you again. I promise!" asserted the Ancient Guru.

The volunteers showered the flower petals on the women. All women were amazed and filled with joy. Something moved within them. They all felt loved and blessed.

"We honor you all, my light warriors, for being here. Your presence in this session proves that you are on the mission to give the best to your baby and the world at large. Congratulations! on being a light warrior," said the Ancient Guru.

Nurture the Nature

Here is your homework. Bring one sapling home and nurture that sapling. No excuses for space, please. Make space for at least one sapling. I am not asking for more. When the sapling grows, you will also grow along with it. You will feel wonderful.

Ananya thought about her terrace. She doesn't have a single plant yet. Arjun loved the plants, but he didn't insist on bringing them home due to work pressure. *Nurturing a plant was too much work so I avoided it. My terrace needs a makeover now.* Ananya mentally made a list of plants she would like to bring home.

"So, even with one sapling at your home, you will feel the peacefulness within you. You might be inspired to bring more plants or make compost at your home. Feel free to explore. Also, those who don't have anyone to share their thoughts can talk with the plants. Its nature's best medicine. This simple activity has cured several diseases which modern science struggles to heal. It is that potent."

Riya thought that she did not need to talk to plants because she had Varun.

It would be a fun activity, Ananya thought.

The Ancient Guru paused, took a breath of fresh, clean air and spoke, "Some of you might think that you don't need to talk to the plants, maybe because you have people to share your thoughts and emotions with or you find it stupid. For the former kind of people, no one on this planet knows you more than you. There are certain things that we can't share with others. Those are our deep secrets. They are part of our souls. You can share those with nature. It will relax you and heal you emotionally. And about stupidity, several experiments[xl] have shown that plants can listen to us and feel our emotions. Trees are excellent listeners and they will respond to you by blossoming completely[xli]."

Riya realized her mistake. *I was being so stubborn. I should try it.*

"Let's now move on to the next ritual. How many of you love to listen to music?" asked the Ancient Guru.

Instantly, 80% of women raised their hands.

"The variety of music can be different. It can be Instrumental, Bollywood songs, Rap songs Sufi, Ghazals, Bhajans, etc., but no person dislikes music. Do we have anyone here?" asked the Ancient Guru.

No one raised their hands.

"Everyone likes some kind of music. Music is connected with our very existence. It's said that the universe was created with a sound and that sound is OM.[xlii] We can say that we were born out of OM and that is why we feel peaceful when we chant OM. Since OM is the basic sound of the universe; chanting it tunes us into the universal frequency and reminds us of our connection to everything in the world[xliii]. After knowing this, we can safely say that **we have music in every cell of our body.**"

 RITUAL #9: Listen To Music Every Day

"Music is a potent tool to get our vibrations in tune with the frequency of the universe. The kind of music you listen to decides what you attract in your life. When people are depressed, they listen to heart-breaking songs and attract more pain in their lives. In contrast, when people listen to positive music, it fills them with positivity. These days we even have music therapy. Has anyone heard about it?" asked the Ancient Guru.

Around 800 women raised their hands.

"Great! It is a different branch of alternative healing. The existence of music therapy is proof of its impact on people across the globe. Music is therapeutic[xliv]. It relaxes the mind and the body. It brings you to the present moment, relieves the stress and makes your life happier," explained the Ancient Guru.

"When you listen to music during your pregnancy, it works on your body and through you on your baby and eases the built-up tension in the body. ***Sow the seeds of good taste for music in your baby.***"

"Whatever you hear during your pregnancy will have impressions in the subconscious mind of your baby and will have an impact throughout his life. Your baby would develop a choice for that kind of music. When you sing the songs, you listened to during your pregnancy to your baby, he will express different emotions and will be able to connect with the music instantly. So, listen to sattvic music, as it invokes positive emotions within you during your pregnancy journey."

"Let's soak in this knowledge for a moment before we move ahead. Relax and close your eyes and take long deep breaths," instructed the Ancient Guru.

Light soothing music was played in the background. There was no other human noise. The windchime bells rang softly and the winds kissed the young mothers. The sound of chirping birds added to the calming effect. A distant sound of the roosters calling could be heard. It was serene and peaceful and the crowd was lost in the magic of music.

After a few minutes, the Ancient Guru said, "Whenever you feel like it, you may gently open your eyes."

Everyone was fresh and childlike again.

"We have discussed the importance of music. Now let's look into what kind of music should be listened to and how we should listen to the music. Don't worry about remembering it. You will be able to recall all that is required to be recalled."

I.   Garbh Sanskar

"Garbh Sanskar music compiles the hymns and chants from the four Vedas – the Rig, Atharva, Yajur and Sama relevant during pregnancy. It covers the preconception phase, womb protection, good health, virtues in baby and delivery. Various religious communities have different compilations that are time-tested and have benefitted several mothers. You can listen to the compilation of your community, or you can listen to the collections of Balaji Tambe, a very famous Garbh Sanskar Guru of western India."

"You must listen to Garbh Sanskar music while seated with your eyes closed and hands on your womb. You can listen to all other kinds of music while sitting or doing various activities by playing it in the background."

"Why Master?" said a woman from the first row with golden hair.

"When you sit in a receptive mode, you and your baby can absorb the energy generated by the chants. Keep your spine erect while listening to it. Through the Sahasrara chakra, universal energy enters your body and travels to your tail bone via the spinal cord. Let me give you an example. If the road isn't open or it's bumpy, isn't it challenging to reach our destination? Similarly, when we keep our spine erect, our body can easily absorb the positive energy in the environment and heal itself. That is why we must keep the spine erect while praying or meditating."

A woman in sky-blue long kurta raised her hand.

The Ancient Guru nodded, permitting her to ask.

"Master, I don't understand the meaning of the chants. Do I need to have a thorough understanding before listening? Or can I just listen without knowing its meaning? Will it still be beneficial?" the woman asked.

"Good question, my light warrior! Mostly, the chants will be in Sanskrit. It's not essential to understand the chants. Whether you know it or not, it will still have its effect. We can take the analogy of food here. We might not know the nutritional value of all the food we eat, but our body will break it down and absorb the nutrients when we eat it. Our knowledge of the nutrients isn't essential for their absorption."

"Similarly, it's not necessary to know the meaning of the chants. If you know it, it's good; if you don't know it, it doesn't matter. All that matters the most is your action. Whether you are listening to it daily and in the manner recommended. This will be your 100% effort, and the rest will be taken care of by the Divine."

II.   Shlokas

"You can listen to any shlokas, chants, strotams, ashtakam, padukas, etc. They are crucial because they will calm you instantly and through you, they will have a calming effect on the baby. Your baby reflects your mood. If you are happy and relaxed, the baby is comfortable and relaxed. If you are in the present moment, the baby is also in the present moment. Whatever you listen to, it will get stored in the subconscious mind of the baby."

But I don't know Sanskrit, Riya thought.

"Most of the Shlokas are in the Sanskrit language. The Sanskrit language aids massively in the development of the baby's mind. It is also used for therapy sessions in psychology and spiritual remissions. The Sanskrit language is so unique that in 1985 Rick Briggs, NASA associate scientist found the Sanskrit language to be most suitable for machine learning and computer programming for artificial intelligence[xlv]," said the Ancient Guru.

"When a mother uses Sanskrit during her pregnancy, the baby's emotional development is tremendous and they are outstanding in the language area. When they grow, they speak clearly, start talking early and have an adorable way of speaking, which attracts people. It also promotes healthy pregnancy," explained the Ancient Guru.

"I do get that most of you might not know Sanskrit. The chants work, whether you know the meaning or not. Yoga works whether you know the benefits or not. The law of gravity works whether you know about it or not. Similarly, Sanskrit works whether you know the basics or not. If you can learn from the basics, it's excellent. Still, in this limited time of just nine months, I understand that doing everything won't be possible. Don't stress out and take baby steps," suggested the Ancient Guru.

Riya was relieved knowing that her baby will benefit from the shlokas despite her not knowing Sanskrit.

HOMEWORK

Shloka Book
I would recommend just writing one shloka every day. Make a Shloka book and write one shloka in it every day. This way, you will have more than 200 shlokas by the end of your pregnancy journey.

"Please don't try to learn them by heart. It's not required. And don't revise them. You don't have to take your test to check how well you remember. Just pick one shloka, learn it, write in your book, and recall it throughout the day. That's it. Then move on to the next shloka the next day. All the warriors who you are going to make the shloka book today can show me a thumbs up."

90% of the women raised their hands and showed thumbs up.

Here are some of the shlokas. They will energize your body and feed your soul. You can even chant them.

    i.   Namaami dhanvantarim aadidevam,
          suraasurair vandita paadapadmam|
          loke jaraaruk bhaya mrityunaasham,
          dhaataaram eesham vividhaushadhinaam ||
   ii.   Aum Tryambakam yajaamahe
          Sugandhim pushtivardhanam |
          Urvaarukamiva bandhanaan
          mrityormuksheeya maamritaat ||
  iii.   Om bhur bhuvaha svaha
          Tat savitur varenyam
          Bhargo devasya dhimahi
          Dhiyo yo nah prachodayat ||

iv. Ya devi sarva bhuteshu, shanti rupena sangsthita
Ya devi sarva bhuteshu, shakti rupena sangsthita
Ya devi sarva bhuteshu, matri rupena sangsthita
Yaa devi sarva bhuteshu, buddhi rupena sangsthita
Namastasyai, namastasyai, namastasyai,
namo namaha | |

v. Karpūragauraṁ karuṇāvatāraṁ, sansārsāram
bhujagendrahāram |
sadāvasantaṁ hṛdayāravinde, bhavaṁ
bhavānīsahitaṁ namāmi | |

vi. Vakratunda Mahakaya, Surya Koti Samaprabaha
Nirvighnam Kurumedeva Sarva Karyeshu Sarvada | |

vii. Sarva maṅgala māṅgalye śhive sarvārthasādhike
śaraṇye tryambake gauri nārāyaṇi namo'stu te | |

viii. Yada yada hi dharmasya, Glanir bhavati bharata
Abhyuthanam adharmasya, Tadaatmaanam
srijaamyaham | |

III. Chants

"You must listen to chants. They are very powerful. They energize the body, mind and soul. Chants help us get above our emotions and live the life of an extraordinary pursuit."

"Let's take an example. Can you recall your mood during the festive times? Don't the festivals energize you? Also, the food made during the festivals has a different taste than that prepared otherwise. That's all because of the energy and our emotions associated with it. The chants fill our hearts with joy and strengthen us from inside out. They generate tremendous energy, which gets stored in food and alters its taste. Also, the Sushumna Nadi gets activated when you listen to certain kinds of music. I would suggest you to listen to one chant every day."

135

IV.   Bhajans

"The next kind of music which you should listen to is devotional songs. In India, most of us listen to them during festivals like Ganesh Chaturthi, Durga Puja, Janmashtami, etc. But typically, we don't listen to them. When you are pregnant, imagine every day to be a festival and festivals are meant to be celebrated. Listen to some bhajans daily. You don't have to set a particular time for it. You can listen to them while traveling, cooking, doing household chores, etc. Bhajans based on ragas work best. They help in the development of the fetus and healthy pregnancy. But if you dislike them after listening 4-5 times, you can skip them. But don't skip them just by listening to them once. Our mind takes time to get habituated to new things. You can skip if you dislike them after five times of listening because it creates negative emotions within you and affects the baby when you do something you dislike. So, don't do anything which you don't like. Don't force yourself too much. It will defeat the whole purpose of Garbh Sanskar. Do you know what is the most important thing to do in Garbh Sanskar? Any guesses?" asked the Ancient Guru.

Music, healthy eating, meditation, etc., were some of the answers.

"We have enthusiastic warriors today!" said the Ancient Guru. "But, you are wrong! the most important thing is to be **HAPPY**. You need to celebrate life to attract an ever-smiling baby. Live life to the fullest and attract an abundance of joy and happiness."

"Now let me see how joyful you are," the Ancient Guru looked at the happy faces of all the women.

The Ancient Guru joined both his hands and clapped thrice. "Clap for yourself, my light warriors. You are strong! You are determined! You are a supermom of this generation!"

The women clapped enthusiastically.

Ananya's eyes sparkled with excitement. She always wanted to bring change in society, but then life happened. She helped people by providing free legal aid, but the reach was limited to just 2-3 people every month. She wanted to impact more lives and now she has got her chance. *By giving my all in, I can finally serve society through my motherhood. I am delighted.*

V. Lullabies

"Lullabies or Lohris are at the very heart of motherhood because babies love lullabies. No digital lohris, please. You might wonder why. Let's take an example. Suppose it's your marriage anniversary. What would you like more? The first option is your husband plays a piece of romantic music on Alexa, phone and anything else and the second option is he prepares a song and especially sings for you no matter how bad he sings," asked the Ancient Guru.

"Sings for me," shouted a lady in a cream jumpsuit.

"Is it the same answer for everyone else too?" asked the Ancient Guru.

"Yes Master," the crowd answered.

"Great! So, do the same for your baby. Say 'NO' to digital lullabies. You need to listen to them and learn them for your baby. Wouldn't you want to give the baby what they like the most? Lohris, baby songs and stories are their favorite things. To become a good mother, you need to know a lot of lullabies, baby songs and stories. Kids love variety and just like any other human being, they will get bored with the same song and that's why you need a lot of them to entertain your baby. Modern mothers don't know lullabies and think they can always play them on some app. But it won't work. It will be very superficial. Imagine you are attending a workshop virtually and you are attending it physically. Which one would you prefer if you get the same speaker in your city? Will your experience be different when you attend it live in your town?" asked the Ancient Guru.

"Yes," a few women answered.

"Another example is homemade food and outside restaurant food. We, as humans, are emotion-driven and are not robots. Our emotions are attached to everything we do. Home-cooked food is full of prana because we cook with love whereas restaurants food is cooked for monetary purposes. So, they contain different emotions. Home-cooked meals satisfy the soul, whereas restaurant food just fills your tummies. Digital Lohris are like restaurant food and in contrast, the lohris sung by you are like homemade food."

"Further, babies listen to lohri when they are about to sleep. That's when their conscious mind rests and subconscious mind activates. So, these lullabies leave deep impressions on your baby's subconscious mind. Be wise in picking lullabies. Select meaningful lohris that describe the qualities you want in your baby. But please don't play it. Just sing them. You can use google to find your choice of music and baby songs. You can learn anything you like. No matter how bad you sing, your emotions while you sing will always be at a much higher level than any famous singer, no matter how good they sing because you will be singing for your baby. The emotions of a mother are very powerful. Your baby will be able to see them in your eyes. He won't just listen to your words while you sing; he will feel the love behind your voice and feel loved and valued."

VI.   Baby Songs

"Baby songs are songs composed especially for babies. You should listen to them in the first four months of your pregnancy and start learning and singing from your fifth month onwards. Do this for both lullabies and baby songs. Baby songs contain the elements that babies love the most. Which elements do you think the babies like the most?"

The answers were train, airplane, sun, moon, animals, birds, nature, festivals, balloons, rain, elephants, cat, dog, etc.

"Wow! You all already know the elements. Baby songs are based on these elements and that is why babies enjoy them a lot. They are loved by all kids alike irrespective of their community or location. So, mothers, you must sing baby songs to your baby. You don't have to allot extra time for it. You can sing while you take your baby for a bath or while cooking or playing with him. Your baby will instantly connect with it and recognize things quickly. Baby songs increase the baby's imaginative power, and sometimes babies start making and singing their versions of songs too. Songs also sharpen their IQ and kindle curiosity within them. They work on all three aspects – IQ, EQ and SQ of the baby. Aren't these reasons enough for you to learn them?"

"Yes," the crowd answered.

"But please don't just play the songs to your baby," requested the Ancient Guru. "You can use google to make the collection that connects most to you and enjoy singing with the baby for the baby's best development."

VII.   Instrumental Music

"Instrumental music has a calming effect on the mind and the body[xlvi]. Various instruments stimulate different chakras, so it's good to listen to instrumental music. You can listen to it while having your tea or doing household and even add them to your meditations. You can pick your choice of instrumental music. All instrumental music is good, but string instrumental music is best for pregnancy. Can you tell me what are string instruments?" asked the Ancient Guru.

Ananya answered, "Guitar."

Another woman said, "Violin."

Some other answers were Sitar, Veena, Banjo, Viola, Harp and Cello.

"Right! the music generated with the use of string is classified as string instrumental music. Choose what touches your heart and make a folder of your favorite instrumental music so that you can listen to them whenever you want."

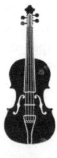

PLAY THE MUSICAL INSTRUMENT
Along with listening to music, I would also recommend you to learn to play any musical instrument. Those who already know can practice what they know in-depth and those who don't know can pick any instrument and learn. Your baby will also learn along with you and will love the sound of the music. Panio is easy, but you are free to choose any other instrument and the sky is the limit.

I would stick to the piano as there is a lot to do in a limited time. Ananya's mind started scanning for the music teacher who could teach her piano.

Riya used to play sitar in her college days. But after marriage and the baby, she hasn't touched it even once. Varun doesn't even know how well she plays. She recalled the old college days and blushed a little on remembering her stage performances during college fests. She made a mental note to take the sitar from her mom's home and play it regularly.

VIII.   Mozart music

"Research has proven that Mozart's music increases spatial reasoning[xlvii]. It works by stimulating the logical mind. So, you can add Mozart music to your daily or weekly routine. However, the key thing here is **engagement** and **enjoyment**. It won't be beneficial if you don't enjoy it. If you dislike it, you can skip it," said the Ancient Guru.

"Please remember not to take the stress. Don't think, 'oh, I have to do this,' 'I have to do that,' 'I don't have time,' etc. Don't get overwhelmed otherwise, the whole purpose will be defeated. You must enjoy whatever you do, or else you will transfer stress and anxiety to your baby. Be easy on yourself. But that doesn't mean you don't do it but enjoy what you do. You don't need to be an expert, so don't seek perfection. Your 100% efforts are more than enough and your baby will be filled with enthusiasm, love and commitment," said the Ancient Guru.

"Now let's discuss our next ritual. The tenth ritual is engaging yourself in creativity – it could be drawing, painting, sketching, stitching, crafting, etc."

 RITUAL #10: Engage Yourself In Creativity

"Any kind of craft leading to creation is incredible. It will stimulate your brain's creative side and send positive signals to the baby. You can even draw mandalas; write a story or a song; or perform a drama. The key is to break your boundaries and come out of your comfort zone. Whatever qualities you have right now will already be transferred to the baby. But we also

141

want the qualities which you don't possess. So, try things you are not confident about and get your breakthroughs."

OPEN A CREATIVE MINI SHOP

My recommendation is to pick one field and instead of just creating a craft and putting it in your wardrobe, try to open your mini online shop and sell your art. You can do that simply by using social media. That will boost your confidence and also keep you engaged in creativity. When you start earning from it, it will motivate you further to continue. While doing it just for yourself, it might become dull after some time. After losing that wow factor, you might leave it altogether. So, open your creative mini shop.

A woman wearing a long black dress asked, "But Master, we won't be able to continue that store after delivery. So why should we open it?"

The Ancient Guru said, "Yes! That's true. We intend to engage in creativity. Still, we don't intend to establish a business here and earn money. Be clear with your intentions and then closing it won't hurt you. Don't get driven by it so much that it starts putting work pressure on you. You have to be as free as a bird. No stress allowed."

A few women clapped, many more joined and soon the park was filled with thunderous applause.

The Ancient Guru spread both his arms at shoulder level and started moving them up and down like the wings of a bird. He asked the crowd to join and soon, all the women spread their wings and dropped off all their inhibitions. They become as free as a bird.

"Now, let's talk about the logical mind. For logical mind stimulation, what should we do? Any guesses?" asked the Ancient Guru.

Ananya answered, "Math?"

"Perfect! I would recommend all of you to learn Vedic math or abacus. Practice it daily for at least ten minutes."

 RITUAL #11: Solve Puzzles Daily

"Math is the easiest and most powerful way to develop logical thinking. It stimulates your left hemisphere and the child will also learn through you. Those who are strong in math during their school days generally make rational decisions in their life," said the Ancient Guru.

"You can solve puzzles, the Rubik's cube, different brainstorming games, etc. Pick your kind of challenge and enjoy it."

Ananya thought about chess. Arjun used to say we shouldn't play chess during pregnancy and focus on other things. Now Ananya got good reasons to play chess. Chess stimulates the logical brain. *We will play chess five days a week*, Ananya declared. She had been playing chess since the age of six. The only good memory she had about her dad was his lessons on the game of chess.

"You can solve sudoku too. Solve a sudoku every day. It can be addictive for many of you. Even I had a hard time leaving the sudoku addiction in my young days," the Ancient Guru chuckled.

Riya was again taken back to her college days. Her friends used to challenge each other to solve sudoku in the fastest time possible. Whoever solved the puzzle first would win and the canteen bill of the winner was on the gang for that day. *Those were fun days.*

"Puzzles will help the baby think logically and question everything. Babies whose logical mind is developed well always do things with reason. Most of the world's successful leaders have a strong rational mind. So, do add some puzzles in your pregnancy journey. I want to add one disclaimer here. Be careful what you wish for. If you want a logical baby, be prepared to answer them. You might feel they are questioning you back. But it might just be that they want to know the reason for doing the things you ask them to do. So, when you want the best baby, you need to be the best first. Consider this, you follow everything and attract the baby of your dreams but then you again go back to your old habits. You won't be able to handle the best baby. That won't be fair to him and will hamper his growth. So, when you wish for a logical baby, you need to keep your mind at a higher consciousness and be ready to nurture a genius mind. Can you all commit?"

"Yes!" the crowd answered enthusiastically.

"Are you capable of nurturing a genius?" asked the Ancient Guru.

"YES!" the women shouted again.

"Great! The next ritual is reading!!! Do you like to read the books?" asked the Ancient Guru.

"No," said the crowd.

RITUAL #12: Feed Your Soul By Reading Books Daily

The Ancient Guru let out a deep breath, "I completely get it that it might be boring for most of you, but there is no choice. Reading books is one of the most powerful habits. Knowledge awakens you and helps you grow. It gives you a new perspective. It deepens your faith in things and sometimes takes you to the fantasy world. Reading a book is like reading the minds of great authors and having a conversation with them over a cup of coffee. When you read autobiographies, you adopt some of the qualities of great legends who were heroes of their times and who brought a revolution in this world. You will start subconsciously thinking and behaving like them. And guess what? These changes will reflect in your baby too. Who doesn't want that?" asked the Ancient Guru.

Have a cup of coffee with Swami Vivekananda! That's interesting. Ananya was an avid reader, but she never looked at reading books in this way.

The Ancient Guru said, "We all have heard this age-old saying:"

'Books are our best friends.'

"Both mother and baby are benefitted tremendously when the mother reads a book."

"If you haven't inculcated a habit of reading yet, motherhood gives you a second chance to grow and expand your mind."

Riya was wearing a yellow suit, long silver jhumkas and red bhindi, resembling a sunflower. She hated reading books. She raised her right hand to ask a question.

145

The Ancient Guru nodded, giving her permission to ask her a question.

"Master, can't we skip reading the books altogether? You told us that we shouldn't force ourselves into something we dislike and skip the bhajans if we don't like it. So, can we do the same with the books?"

The Ancient Guru raised both hands and clapped. "Excellent question! I am sorry for those amongst you who don't like to read. I can't permit you to skip reading books. In the Music section too, you can search and make your playlist, but don't skip music altogether. It's the same for books. You can make your list of books. You can start by reading on topics which interest you. But you can't skip reading altogether."

"There are certain skills that are life-supporting. For example, everyone needs to know how to cook. Even though you can hire someone to cook for you, you must still know because they might take leaves. You don't want your family to eat unhealthy restaurant food for many days. Also, a pandemic can happen, and you might find yourself in the kitchen. I even consider swimming a life-saving skill. Only if everyone knew how to swim, no one in the world would die by drowning."

"Even if you don't like to cook, you need to cultivate your interest in cooking because it's essential for you and your family's health. For all the life-supporting skills, you need to put conscious efforts to inculcate them. You don't like it because you aren't habituated to it since childhood. Right now, you have a miracle chance to break your old patterns and become your best version. There is no other way. It's the same for those who dislike meditating. It's also a life-supporting skill you must know and practice, at least during pregnancy. Doing meditation is one of the easiest ways to relieve stress and be in the present moment. It won't come in your baby if you don't

146

do it. So, forget your likes and dislikes and take a leap of faith and do it. Trust the universe and it will always guide you to become your best version."

"Any ritual is challenging to begin, chaotic in the middle but fantastic at the end. Reading a book requires the same discipline, as taking care of a sapling or learning a musical instrument, or solving sudoku. It's that unavoidable ritual without which your pregnancy journey would be incomplete. The books fill in the gaps. They empower you. They broaden your thinking and they become part of your soul. So, read the book and sprinkle the knowledge on your baby. His mind will expand tremendously."

"When you put in the efforts to learn any skill, many changes happen at a cellular level in your body. When you start the learning process, your baby will also learn to put in the effort to develop new habits. Otherwise, he might leave things with slight discomfort. We would never want our kids to leave the formal education. Isn't it compulsory to take formal education?" asked the Ancient Guru.

"Yes," the crowd replied collectively.

"Why?" asked the Ancient Guru playfully.

For a better future, for knowledge, for a better life, for a job, to become successful, etc. were some of the answers.

"Exactly! Formal education plays a very important role in the baby's development. Similarly, all the life-supporting skills have a crucial role in one's life."

"Wow!" a few women from the second row exclaimed. Many women applauded cheerfully.

The Ancient Guru paused, moving his neck up and down, and pulled back his shoulders. He closed his eyes for a second and took a deep breath. "Let me tell you how you should do every activity. Do your work with 100% attention. When you do a particular work, don't think of anything else. Be there. Live that moment. It will give you immense peace. People these days hardly live in the present moment. They are constantly running from one thing to another. This exhausts them physically and mentally. Their minds either run in the future or get stuck in the past. When you bring it to the present moment, you feel peaceful and don't feel an energy drain. Do your work with utmost focus and keep your mind powerful. When it goes somewhere else, gently bring it back to the work you are doing. When you are completely into the activity, your state of mind will be different. You will resonate at a frequency closer to that of the universe. Further, take full responsibility. The more responsibilities you take, the stronger you will become. It will increase your confidence and capacity to get things done. But don't forget to enjoy what you do and live your life to its fullest potential," the Ancient Guru concluded energetically.

"Are you all ready to read the books now?" asked the Ancient Guru.

The crowd answered affirmatively.

"Let's look at the kind of books that are beneficial for you and your baby."

1   Self-development books

"The first category includes those books that will help you grow. They will change the way you think and help you develop healthy habits. We all are here to become our best versions and the self-help books are one of the most crucial tools in our self-development journey."

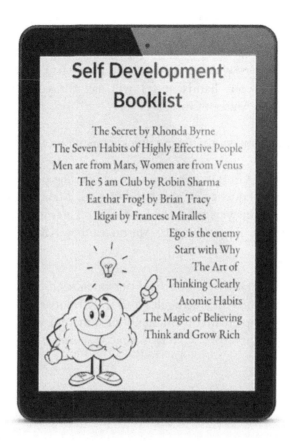

"The first recommended book on the list is 'The Secret'. It will help you to understand the rules of manifestation. The second book will make you a more efficient person and those qualities will be transferred to your baby. The third book is for a healthy married life. The relationship between the husband and the wife has a profound impact on the baby. Researches have shown that only a good husband and wife can become good parents[xlviii]. Through this book, couples can understand their partners. Couples can step into each other's shoes and enhance understanding between them to reduce conflicts and create that magical bond of love. You can pick any book from the self-help genre."

2   Autobiographies

"The second category is autobiographies. Let's play a game. Name a person who inspires you the most. It will be a rapid game. Raise your hands and I will ask for your answer," explained the Ancient Guru.

The enthusiastic women were quickly raising their hands.

The Ancient Guru made eye contact, giving permission to answer in a sequence of the hands raised. Mahatma Gandhi was the first answer, followed by Mother Teresa, Elon Musk, Bhagat Singh, Abdul Kalam, Martin Luther King, Abraham Lincoln, etc.

"Great! We all know about these personalities, but it's time to look deeper into their struggles and their mindset. When you read with complete involvement about someone, you pick their qualities subconsciously. Here is a recommended list:"

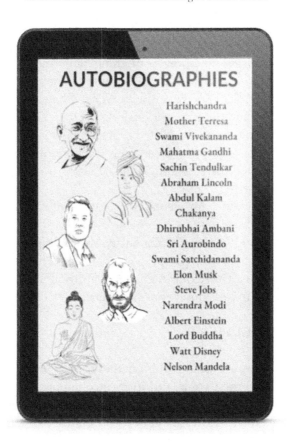

"My light warriors, audiobooks are best to be avoided," declared the Ancient Guru.

"Why Master?" a woman from the fourth row asked.

"While you read, your 100% focus is on reading, but it's not the same in audiobooks. When you listen to an audio or watch a movie, it's a passive activity. In contrast, when you read books, it's an active activity. Your mind doesn't stay there. It thinks of several different activities while you are still watching the movie or listening to the book. You can't do the same while you read the book because if you do, you won't be able to

151

understand what's written. You don't just read words; you read the emotions and visualize the things. You stay in the present moment; you get to know something new and you attract growth. You get a sense of accomplishment when you complete a book. They have the power to change you. When you listen to audiobooks, you stay distracted. You focus less and your mind wanders. You hardly remain in the present moment. So, will you avoid the audiobooks, my light warriors?" asked the Ancient Guru.

"Yes," a few women answered. Some of them nodded.

"Stay with good books. Have a coffee with Gandhi and other great personalities from pre-pregnancy till delivery to make you a better person. Those books change your thoughts and habits and help you in becoming your best version."

3. Garbh Sanskar

"The next genre is reading about the Garbh Sanskar. Doing this will strengthen your faith in the technique and motivate you to stay committed to your rituals. Trust is important to keep things moving. Reading books on Garbh Sanskar will do that for you. Suggestions:"

i.   Balaji Tambe's Ayurvedic Garbh Sanskar
ii.   Garbh Sanskar by Suresh Alka

"I found these two original books in English. Don't read all the books in this genre, as it might confuse you. Read only the authentic books."

Ananya and a few other women were making notes on their mobile phones.

The Ancient Guru noticed it and said, "I would like to share with you what my mentor had shared with me. During my college days, we had a few lectures by honorary faculties. I used to make notes of whatever the faculty taught in all the classes, and they encouraged it. But, one of the honorary faculties had a unique style of teaching. He asked everyone to put the pen down. If any of the students picked up a pen to write, the faculty would stop teaching. Everyone in the class was surprised."

The topper of the class asked, "Sir, if we don't write, how will we remember it?"

The faculty answered, "Trust me! If you listen to whatever I teach with your 100% attention, you will be able to remember it. I don't think it will be required, but still, I will give you five minutes extra at the end of the class to note down the important points and ask me if you forget anything. But during the class, I don't want anyone of you to write. When you have a pen in your hand, your 80% focus is on writing rather than listening and understanding things. In my class, we will focus on listening and understanding the concepts. And once you know the concepts, there is no way you can forget them."

"This is what I learned from my mentor and I teach the same to my students," shared the Ancient Guru proudly.

The women immediately stopped making notes on their mobile phones. Ananya felt embarrassed and realized her mistake too. She quickly kept her phone aside.

4. Contemporary Fiction/Story Books

"The next category is story books. This category will help you escape from reality, break your monotonous routine and strengthen your imaginative ability."

Riya's eyes twinkled on listening to this category. Stories always fascinated her. She was a die-hard fan of marvel and read

153

comics during her college days. *I would read all marvel comics in the market as soon as they would come.*

"Those who dislike reading books can start by reading story books. These books will take you to different places and mesmerize you with their beauty. It cultivates imagination and you are able to travel virtually anywhere. It gives you an easy escape from the routine. When you read a book about a fantasy world, your baby also travels with you. Make sure you read stories of courage. Through them, you can inculcate the virtue of courage within you and your baby. Further, you can read literary works with vivid descriptions of scenes and situations to get a new perspective. You will learn to find beauty in everything. Wouldn't you like that your baby finds beauty in everything?"

Without waiting for the answer, the Ancient Guru continued, "Let's take an example. When you buy a dress, you feel it's a fabulous dress. But do you think the same every time you take it out from your wardrobe?"

"No," the crowd answered.

"That's because we take it for granted. We don't value it after we possess it and the WOW factor is lost. However, babies find the WOW factor in anything and everything. They collect the stones, play with flowers, leaves, sand, water puddles, and other things that we as adults ignore. This quality keeps them happy and our indifference keeps us stressed and unhappy."

The crowd was amazed by how easily and effectively the Guru had put forward this life-changing knowledge.

"Try to develop this quality. It will give you everlasting happiness and satisfaction. It would be great if you try to bring the WOW factor into your life. It keeps up the enthusiasm and you stay away from negative thoughts. **It brings more life to your life,"** suggested the Ancient Guru.

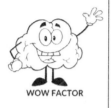

WOW FACTOR

WOW MOMENTS

The more AHA moment you bring to your day, the more you stay happy and in the present moment. With practice, you can develop this quality of being surprised and appreciating everything in your life. Here is what you need to do. Every week pick one day and on that day find 24 AHA moments - One for each hour. You need to say WOW aloud 24 times on that day. Gradually it will become a part of your nature.

"We can't change the situation, but we can change how we look at it. We can change ourselves and then the problem loses its power. Read books about fairy tales, magical places and wonderlands. Through such books, your baby will develop a very high emotional and spiritual quotient. The highest level of spirituality is finding this wow factor. That is one of the things we try to achieve through meditation. The other way is through reading the books."

"Stories have moral values. It's easier to understand the values through stories. Kids love stories. Reading a storybook also prepares you to tell the stories to your baby later. You will know what to say and you can even write your own stories. It will strengthen ethics in you. Keep some short books for the 9th month as they are exciting and you can escape from your physical discomfort through them. They are light reads and will entertain you while you relax on your couch with that big belly in the 9th month. Here is the sample book list:"

1   House on the harbor
2   Lighthouse on the lake
3   The elephant vanishes
4   Wise and otherwise

5   The Greatness Guide
6   The Seven Habits of Happy Kids
7   Grandma's bag of stories
8   Panchatantra stories
9   Ramayana
10 Mahabharata
11 Ruskin bond books
12 Akbar and Birla
13 Vikram Bethal stories
14 Chacha Chaudhary
15 Tenali Raman
16 Sinhasan Battisti
17 Shakuntala by Kalidasa
18 Meghdut by Kalidasa
19 Chicken soup for soul booklets (9th month)

"Further, you can read any books of interest except murder mysteries, news and those which involve negative things. The news mainly contains negative incidents. Reading about them makes the baby feel unsafe. They send negative emotions. For some of you, avoiding news reading might be difficult. If it's crucial, you can request your friends or family to filter out information and tell you only the positive news such as new laws, judgments, scientific research, etc."

"Reading is a lifelong process. Don't leave your new friends – your books. Post-delivery pick parenting books. Don't leave them if you want to continue growing and evolving in life."

"Do you want to know more?" asked the Ancient Guru.

"Yes," replied half of the crowd.

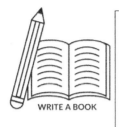

WRITE A BOOK

> ## BECOME AN AUTHOR
> Like I suggested to open your creative shop online; similarly, you can even write a book during your pregnancy and become a published author. Wouldn't it be great? You don't need to have mastery in any particular field; you can just write a novel or a novella or a storybook for kids. Later read that book to your baby. He will surely be very proud of you.

The crowd was surprised by the Ancient Guru's idea. The eyes of a few women widened.

It's a fantastic suggestion, Ananya thought.

Riya had already started making plans to write a storybook for kids. The stories have a special place in her heart. They connect her with her soul.

"Loved the idea, right?" asked the Ancient Guru.

"Yes," the crowd answered enthusiastically.

The Ancient Guru said, "You all have grown tremendously in the last few days. Keep this enthusiasm alive and become your best version. Don't forget to do your homework today. We will have the last session tomorrow. There is a surprise for you. Those who have pets at home can bring them here and volunteers will take care of them."

Everyone clapped for the Master and rejoiced. Few women even stood up and the rest followed. Light music was played by one of the volunteers in the background and the women started moving their hands from right to left, then left to right over their heads. They all were dancing with joy. They all knew that they wouldn't have ever thought about the things shared by the Master. Their old self wasn't capable of doing these

157

things. They weren't their old self anymore. They had grown. They had gained immense wisdom in the last six days. They were stronger. They now had a community that had their back if they fell.

After a few minutes, the music was stopped. The Ancient Guru felt happy seeing the vigor of the crowd.

"Sangachadwam."

The Ancient Guru joined his hands in namaste mudra, bowed his head, and left the stage.

Ananya and Riya looked at each other and hugged instantly. "I will write a book," both said at the same time.

"Wow," again both spoke at the same time.

"Congratulations!" again at the same time and they laughed.

"This calls for a celebration," asserted Ananya.

"Definitely. But where?" asked Riya.

"Beach party with husbands this evening?" suggested Ananya

"That would be perfect!" exclaimed Riya.

"See you at 6 p.m.," confirmed Ananya.

Riya nodded.

They hugged and bid goodbye and left the park.

A few hours later

Ananya wore a short floral dress with a pearl necklace and studs for the party. She complemented it with Hawaiian slippers. Arjun was on time to pick Ananya up at 5:30 pm at the main gate of their building. Arjun made fun of her slippers because they looked a little childish, but she loved them for their comfort. He was wearing a grey tee with cream colored shorts. He complimented Ananya and then they drove to the rock café, their usual hang-out place on the beach.

As they entered the café, they saw Riya and Varun sitting at the table facing the vastness of the Arabian sea. She felt nostalgic. She loved the magnificence of the ocean and the music was terrific. Ladies decided to have the lemon juice. Arjun settled with a cold coffee. Varun drank occasionally, but today, he took a soda as he had to drive back home.

After the initial chit-chat and drinks, Ananya suggested that they play 'Jenga'. Everyone agreed and Arjun asked the waiter to bring the game to their table.

A few moments later, Jenga blocks were on their table and they started building the tower. After the tower was built, Ananya declared that she would begin first as her name starts with "A." Riya grinned; and Arjun and Varun agreed.

She carefully removed the middle block and it read, "Take dare from the person sitting to your right."

Varun was sitting to her right. He wore a blue shirt and grey chinos. She showed it to him.

Varun read it and dared Ananya to propose to Arjun on one knee.

Ananya rolled her eyes. She wasn't expecting that.

She thought for a moment and smiled. She gently picked up a red rose from the table décor and stood up. She held Arjun's hand gently and he stood up in reflex.

She kneeled and asked, "Will you always be by my side no matter what?" offering the red rose to him.

Arjun and Riya were surprised. Varun gave an appreciative nod.

"Yes, my love! I will always be by your side come what may," said Arjun, gently pulling her up towards him and hugging her. Ananya blushed.

The crowd at the café clapped joyfully.

Then Ananya and Arjun settled on their chairs.

Now it was Arjun's turn to remove the block from the tower. It read, "Would you like to spend your next life with your current partner?"

Everyone made an "Oooooooo" sound.

Arjun thought for a moment and said, "That's a tricky question." Arjun chuckled. "I would love to spend my next life with Ananya with the change of role. I would like to be her and she would step into my shoes. That way it would be more fun."

Ananya made faces. She looked adorable when she did it.

Varun laughed.

Riya played with her long white earrings, which perfectly complemented her halter-necked sky-blue dress and ankle-length faux leather boots. She was next to remove the block. It read, "Do you secretly admire someone other than your partner?"

Varun's eyes broadened.

Riya laughed and confidently answered, "No! the only admiration in my life is Varun".

Ananya gave a high-five. Arjun gave a thumbs-up.

Varun removed the block carefully. The towered shook a little, but he did not let the tower fall. It read, "Take a dare from your partner."

Varun looked at Riya.

"Riya, can I give the dare if you don't mind?" Arjun interrupted.

"Of course, go ahead," Riya answered.

"Bring that hat from the woman sitting at the fourth table in dark green dress for free," dared Arjun.

"How can I do that?" Varun asked.

"That's the challenge," Arjun replied playfully, turning his shoulders outwards.

Varun shrugged his shoulders.

He walked towards the woman, picking a carnation flower from the table decor on the way. He chit-chatted for a while and came back with the hat on his head.

Riya whistled.

All the eyes were on her. Many people grinned from ear to ear. The lady whose hat Varun had brought started laughing.

"How did you manage that?" Ananya asked.

"That's a secret," Varun grinned. *I complimented her looks and her dress after giving her the flower. Then I explained to her that we were playing a game and she gave her hat happily.*

They played one more round of Jenga and later, the couples stood up for some dance. A French romantic song was playing in the background. Ananya and Riya were enjoying the moment.

Ananya spotted a tattoo artist and asked if anyone was interested. Riya hopped with her; Arjun and Varun sat near the shore. Ananya chose the hope bird tattoo for her left wrist. In contrast, Riya chose a baby tattoo on her right upper arm. It was a temporary tattoo that would stay for a week.

Later they joined the men and enjoyed the breeze kissing their faces, the smell of the ocean, the melody of waves crashing on the shore and moonlight illuminating their faces. *The day was well spent*, Ananya said to herself.

The vastness of the ocean reminded Ananya of the Ancient Guru and she couldn't help but think about the sessions and what they had learned today. She discussed the day's session with Riya and the genres in which they will be writing their books.

"I think we should make a note of things to be done so that we don't forget anything," suggested Riya.

Ananya agreed and quickly made the to-do list on her mobile.

✏️ TO-DO LIST

1. Make a list of activities you will be doing during your pregnancy.
2. Make a timetable and devote a particular time to each activity. When you do the same activity every day at the same time, it gets established within you faster and reaps you more benefits.
3. If you plan to start your creative business, select your interest area and make the roadmap.
4. If you plan to write a book, think about genre and the deadline for publishing.
5. Make your booklist ready in a week.
6. Create your music folder in a week
7. Choose the musical instrument you will learn during your pregnancy.

Don't get overwhelmed. Do one thing at a time and while doing a particular thing, forget about the rest of the homework. That will keep you calm and you will be able to make wise choices.

DO IT RIGHT

1. Nature is the mother of creativity, just like necessity is the mother of invention.
2. Music is connected with our very existence.
3. When we chant OM, we vibrate at the universal frequency found in all things throughout the universe.
4. When you listen to music during your pregnancy, it works on your body and through you on your baby and eases the built-up tension in the body. Sow the seeds of good taste for music in your baby.
5. When you sing the songs, you listened to during your pregnancy to your baby, he will express different emotions and will be able to connect with the music instantly
6. Shlokas, chants, strotams, ashtakam, padukas, etc., are crucial because they will calm you instantly and through you, they will have a calming effect on the baby.
7. When a mother uses Sanskrit during her pregnancy, the baby's emotional development is tremendous and they are outstanding in the language area
8. Avoid digital lullabies. The baby won't be able to connect with them.
9. The emotions of a mother are very powerful. Your baby will be able to see them in your eyes. He won't just listen to your words while you sing; he will feel the love behind your voice and feel loved and valued.
10. Whatever qualities you have right now will already be transferred to the baby. Try to inculcate the qualities which you don't possess.
11. Math is the easiest and most powerful way to develop logical thinking.
12. Puzzles will help the baby think logically and question everything.
13. Reading books is one of the most powerful habits.

14. Any ritual is challenging to begin, chaotic in the middle but fantastic at the end.
15. The books fill in the gaps. They empower you. They broaden your thinking. And they always become part of your soul.
16. Avoid audiobooks because its passive activity. In contrast, reading a book is an active activity.
17. Bring more WOW factor into your life. It brings more life to your life. It keeps up the enthusiasm and you stay away from negative thoughts.
18. Avoid reading murder mysteries, news and those which involve negative things. They invoke negative emotions.

CHAPTER 9
GARBH SAMVAD

It was the last day of the mastery sessions. Ananya didn't want to be late today. Ananya was talking with her newly bought saplings. She enjoyed talking with the plants. She was amazed by how light she felt after sharing her thoughts with them.

As she sat in her car to drive to the park, she felt a rush of emotions. *I will miss these sessions. Today I am feeling so excited to know about the Ancient Guru. The old lady had promised she will reveal his story to me.* She was thinking about how these sessions had impacted her life. *I have grown tremendously in these six days. I feel more positive, loved and blessed and I am hardly stressed or angry these days.*

Ananya reached the park and again noticed that super-luxury car. It made her wonder about its owner. She was wearing a peacock printed shirt and sky-blue chinos. Her thoughts were interrupted by a light sound coming from the park. At first, she thought she was just imagining things but she knew it was real once she came closer to the class. The Ancient Guru and the volunteers were on stage and light music was playing in the background. She joined the other equally surprised women.

Ananya couldn't find Riya in the session. *She might be late because of the beach party last night,* Ananya thought.

The Ancient Guru greeted everyone with a good morning and asked them to stand at their places and dance to their heart's fill.

"Ooooo!" exclaimed a few women in realization.

Some of the volunteers, ten women wearing yellow sarees and six men wearing brown kurtas along with the Ancient Guru in maroon kasaya, were on the stage. The volume of the music was increased and they started dancing gently.

Ananya was wondering about Riya and just then, Riya tapped her right shoulder. Ananya was relieved.

Ananya scolded Riya for being late and Riya apologized. They also started dancing to the sound of the music. Ananya and Riya had not heard this kind of music before. *I will ask for this soundtrack*, Ananya thought.

The Ancient Guru instructed, "Those who feel like it may close their eyes and surrender themselves completely and sway with the music. Don't resist it. The music can touch the deepest portions of the soul where nothing else can reach. Try to feel the sensations in your body and let the energy flow freely. Surrender completely."

The women followed meekly.

After a few minutes, the music was stopped and the Ancient Guru directed everyone to settle down, close their eyes and take long deep breaths.

"Inhale from the nose and exhale from the mouth. Relax completely."

After a few moments, the Ancient Guru said softly, "whenever you feel complete, you may gently open your eyes."

All the women were filled with gratitude. They felt delighted by the beautiful experience.

The Ancient Guru said, "As we all have already experienced, dance invokes energy within us. Dance helps to release stress and stay happy and relaxed. Through dance, you can revitalize your body and have a healthy pregnancy."

"All our traditional dances invoke this kind of energy within the doer. We all know about the famous tandava. But obviously, that's not recommended for pregnant ladies as that dance form requires tremendous power."

"Pregnant mothers can do light dance just like we did today whenever they feel like doing it. It will take all the stress away."

"Have you all brought your pets to the session?" asked the Ancient Guru.

Around 70 women raised their hands.

The pets were being taken care of by the volunteers. There were 45 dogs, 18 cats, two tortoises and four love birds.

"Oh, the volunteers already took them for the playful walk. That's why I couldn't listen to their sounds. It's okay. I will meet them when they return from their walk," declared the Ancient Guru.

Ananya always thought that keeping pets was too much work. Arjun agreed. So, they never had pets.

"Your pets love when you talk to them, isn't it?" asked the Ancient Guru. "It's one of the most cherished times of their day."

"Yes!" the women with the pets answered collectively.

"Similarly, your baby loves when you talk with him[xlix]. Everyone likes to be spoken to. Your baby loves your attention. Don't you like the attention of your husband and your loved ones?" asked the Ancient Guru.

"Yes, Master!" the crowd answered.

"A baby also craves attention and love. This brings me to today's topic of '**Garbh Samvad**[i].' It simply means talking to your baby. When you talk to your baby, he feels loved and valued. He will develop a healthy emotional quotient and will be full of love."

 ### RITUAL #13: Talk To Your Baby Daily

"For those who find it difficult to talk with the baby in the womb, put your baby in all the roles. Make him your best friend, your brother, your sister, your father, a friend, and sometimes even a guru. In this way, you won't have limited topics to talk about. Talk about anything and everything. This will fill him with lots of love. We want to fill the baby with so much love that he never feels a lack of love. But avoid complaints and negative talks. When you complain and criticize, it drains your energy. You should refrain from complaints in general and avoid complaints or talking about negative things with the baby in Garbh Samvad completely."

"How many of you have done that rice jar experiment[ii] which I gave on the first day?" asked the Ancient Guru.

Around 500 women raised their hands.

"What was the outcome?" enquired the Ancient Guru.

A woman in a magenta jumpsuit answered, "the jar with the grateful tag was not spoiled. The other two jars were spoilt."

"Congratulations! for doing this experiment. Those who have missed it can start today itself. The jar with the hate tag must be in terrible shape, with rice being most decomposed. The neutral jar would be unaffected, and the jar with the gratitude tag would be the healthiest. Our words have power. They transmit energy. You must be very careful about what you share through your words. Don't talk about negative things with your baby. We don't want to transmit negativity to him. The rice jar experiment shows the tremendous impact of words on everything. So, watch your words, my light warriors."

The Ancient Guru paused. The sounds of barking dogs were audible now. The Ancient Guru saw the pets and smiled. He signaled the volunteers to offer food to the pets and they did the needful.

"Due to lifestyle changes and technological advancements, we are more connected than ever yet we've become more distant from each other. People are suffering from mental illnesses. There is a lack of self-love and we harbor chaos instead of peace within us. Only when a person feels full of love, can he share the love with others. One can only share what they have in abundance and not when they lack it," said the Ancient Guru.

"Through these simple talks with the baby, you can fill him with lots of love, care and happiness. Tell him that you love him, that you are excited for him, that you are waiting for him. That you have done all the preparations for his welcome. Speak your heart without filters. Through Garbh Samvad, you can nurture a deeper bond with your baby."

GARBH SAMVAD
Talk to your baby for at least 10 minutes every day. You can start talking whenever you feel like but from the fifth month onwards, add it to the daily routine. This alone has tremendous benefits.

"Some of you might find it challenging to talk aloud with the baby, but it's an important activity. So those who find it difficult can start with shower talk. You can begin by telling the baby that we will take a bath now. We are enjoying the shower. Then you can share your routine with him. Ex. when you eat, you can talk with him. You can say food gives you so many nutrients. **Your baby will feel connected with you for a lifetime with these simple yet powerful activities.** Share with him what you enjoy. Share positive things with him. Just speak it out."

"Further in your ninth month, you can add that soon you will be coming into this world. And you are waiting to welcome him with open arms. This will signal him that people are waiting for him and that the womb isn't his permanent home. This affirmation helps in normal delivery. Also, practice Apana mudra in your 9th month to activate Apana vayu."

"So, who is going to start Garbh Samvad from today?" asked the Ancient Guru.

Around 70% of the crowd raised their hands.

MARMA THERAPY

"Amazing! My light warriors, are you ready for more?" asked the Ancient Guru.

"Yes," the crowd answered in unison.

"We all already know that everything is energy. Let's now learn how to channel this abundance of universal energy to certain parts of the body for healing ourselves completely. There is an ancient therapy in Ayurveda that works on energy points in our body. Our body has thousands of energy points, but 107 points are classified as major energy points[lii]. By stimulating these energy points gently, all the blockages in that region are

171

removed and prana begins to flow freely again. This ancient therapy is called the **Marma therapy**[liii] and the energy points are called the **Marma points**. I know some of you might find it hard to believe this, but it works like magic. Marma therapy has been practiced in ancient India since time immemorial. But, like many other techniques, it is being forgotten with time."

"Marma therapy has tremendous benefits. But if you can't connect with it, you can skip it during your pregnancy. It's our only optional ritual because faith plays a crucial role in its effectiveness," explained the Ancient Guru.

'The Marma therapy is so powerful that it works even in those conditions in which allopathy fails to provide a cure[liv]. It works on our subtle body, which provides energy to our gross/physical body. Some of the examples of marma which we still follow are[lv]:"

1. **Blessing someone:** Positive energy is transferred when you touch the head to bless someone.
2. **Peacock feathers:** Some saints use peacock feathers to bless and heal people. It is also marma as peacock feather stimulates the marma points and removes blockages in the head region.
3. **Wrestling warm-up:** The wrestlers pat their inner thighs and biceps before beginning the match. Stimulating those points increases the oxygen in the body and prepares the body for the energy-intensive activity.
4. **Self-defense[lvi]:** The knowledge of marma is so deep that you can make another person unconscious when you press a particular point. This technique has been applied in martial arts and self-defense.
5. **Namaste:** In India, we greet namaste by joining hands and don't shake the hands or hug. Our leaders were very well aware of the energy exchanges through

marma points. That is why they greeted namaste to avoid an unwarranted exchange of energies through handshakes or hugs.

The Ancient Guru paused and looked at the confused faces of everyone. "I request anyone of you to come here on the stage to experience the magic of this ancient therapy."

Ananya raises her hand first.

The Ancient Guru asked her to come on stage and sit on the chair. He instructed her to close her eyes and relax completely. The Ancient Guru chanted a few mantras and gently touched where her chakras were located, starting from the Muladhara chakra. He placed the first finger of his right hand on her tail bone and moved it gently in a circular motion clockwise and then anti-clockwise three times. After a minute, he moved to the Svadisthan chakra; he repeated the same circular motion and then placed his first finger of the right hand on the Manipur chakra on her spine. Then he moved to the Anahata chakra. He was covering the entire backbone of Ananya. A few moments later, he moved to the Vishuddha chakra. Then he came in front of Ananya and placed the first finger of his right hand on Ajna chakra, between the eyebrows and moved it in a circular motion. After taking a few deep breaths, the Ancient Guru opened up his palms wide and placed them over Ananya's head, covering her entire scalp.

Ananya loved every second of the therapy. She was deeply engrossed with the prana. She couldn't even feel where the touch was made until the palms were placed on her head. She felt as if a divine golden light was flowing through her body. There were no traces of negative emotions such as stress, anxiety, worry, or need for success. No desires, no wants. She was totally in the present moment with an abundance of prana flowing in her body. She was overflowing with positivity. She felt free. She looked radiant. Even the crowd could notice it.

After a few minutes, the Ancient Guru blessed Ananya and asked her to open her eyes gradually.

Ananya didn't wish to open her eyes. She wanted to stay in that state of mind, but she knew she had to. She opened her eyes gently and saw the Master. She thanked him by joining her hands and bowing down.

The Ancient Guru asked her to share her experience with the rest of the crowd.

Ananya stood up from the chair. She took the mic from the volunteer and said, "This was pure magic. I don't know how it works, but it does. I couldn't even feel my existence. I experienced transcendence. I was entirely in some other world. It was heavenly."

"WOW!" expressed some of the women.

The Ancient Guru asked Ananya to go back to her seat.

"So, here was a demonstration of the Marma therapy. Would you like to learn it?"

"Yes," the crowd shouted enthusiastically. Some women in the fourth row whispered that they should have raised their hands.

"But before we learn it, let's look at restrictions first."

1. In this therapy, there is no application of force. The touch is very gentle, just like you touch a newborn baby.
2. The fingers shouldn't be pointed but flat. A pointed finger can hurt.
3. A pregnant woman cannot give this therapy to anyone else because a lot of energy is exchanged at a subtle

level. You can take the therapy from someone who is not pregnant.

4. It's beneficial and safe for a pregnant woman to practice the therapy on herself.

5. It's good to practice the therapy when your stomach is empty for profound effects.

6. While you touch the marma points with the first finger of the right hand, place your left hand in Gyan mudra."

"Do you have any doubts about the restrictions?" asked the Ancient Guru.

"Can we practice the therapy on the baby?" asked a woman from the second row.

The Ancient Guru was happy with this question, "Yes! It will help immensely in his development if you give marma to your baby but first, let's learn to give it to yourself. Become an expert in it and then you can give it to anyone in your family and friends."

 RITUAL #14: Give Yourself Marma Daily

"The Marma therapy is our last ritual. Now let's practice. Keep your eyes closed for the next ten minutes and open them only if you feel necessary. Just follow my instructions. The woman who came for the therapy on stage can avoid doing it and just observe the steps for the home practice."

MARMA PRACTICE

Relax completely. Take a few long, deep breaths. Place the first finger of your right hand between your eyebrow and left hand in Gyan Mudra. Take five long deep breaths. Now place both the palms on the sides of your temples, with fingers pointing up towards the sky. Move your palms in a circular motion clockwise three times and then anti-clockwise three times and stay there. Keep breathing. After 3-5 breaths, place both hands on your ears, fingers pointing towards the back. Be very gentle. Don't apply pressure on your ears. Cover your ears completely. Enjoy the silence and be with your inner voice. Take 3-5 deep breaths. Now place your left hand on your knee in Maha mudra and make a flower with your right hand joining the tips of your finger and thumb and place it on the top of your head on the Sahasrara chakra. Take a few long, deep breaths. Gently place your right palm on your abdomen and left palm below the right palm covering your abdomen completely. Feel as if you are blessing the baby. Take long, deep breaths. After you take five deep breaths, you may relax your hands. But keep your eyes closed and let the prana flow in your body. Feel the sensations in your body. Relax completely.

The young mothers were completely engrossed in the tremendous energies generated in the park. The park was filled with divine prana. There were no lines of stress on their forehead. Through them, even their babies felt calm and relaxed.

After a few minutes, the Ancient Guru instructed softly, "Whenever you feel like you may gently open your eyes."

"How are you feeling, my light warriors? Energetic, right? You can show me a thumbs up," said the Ancient Guru.

"Yes!" the crowd said softly and all of them showed thumbs up. They were still in that meditative state of mind.

MARMA EVERYDAY

These are the five most powerful marma points. Stay at each marma point for 5-10 deep breaths and you can cover them in 10 minutes. Do it daily and you will notice many changes in your life and you will be able to heal yourself completely.

"This was the last session of our workshop, my enthusiastic mothers. It was a wonderful journey with all of you. I hope you were able to discover a new dimension to life. Give your all to implement these lifestyle changes for the best development of your baby. **Garbh Sanskar is not easy, but it's the right thing to do.** Always remember your baby will be what you are 1000x multiplied. Become your best version and give birth to a baby who can impact the whole world and work towards the betterment of society. The future of our planet is in your hands, my light warriors. We have a small gift for all of you. It will remind you of this journey and help you to stay on this path."

"I wish you all the best for your journey. In case you need any guidance during your journey, you can always reach out to our volunteers, and they will help you in every way possible."

"Sangachadwam."

The Ancient Guru showed a thumbs up to the crowd, blessed everyone and left the stage.

The volunteers distributed the gift. It was a statue of a mother holding her baby in her arms and sitting under a huge tree. The mother's face was calm and peaceful. It was the perfect gift for light warriors.

Riya and Ananya loved the gift. Riya said, "I will keep it on the side table in my bedroom so that it reminds me of these sessions every morning."

Ananya said, "That's perfect! I will keep it on my office table so that I can keep stress at bay."

Both of them decided to start practicing rituals from the next day onwards at Ananya's house. Riya hugged Ananya and left the park.
Ananya went to meet the old lady after the session. She was waiting for Ananya as promised. She offered Ananya herbal tea and some snacks.

"So young lady, tell me what do you want to know?" asked the old one.

Ananya thanked her for the snacks and asked, "why is the Ancient Guru on this path? What motivates him? Where is his family and what does he do for a living as these sessions are free?"

"So, you want to know everything!" the old lady laughed.

"He is a genius, comes from wealth, is a philanthropist and runs several schools and NGOs."

Ananya was surprised to hear this. *If he is so rich and busy, why does he hold sessions on Garbh Sanskar?*

"Money never gave him peace and satisfaction. He always wanted the best for everyone. Improving others' lives gave him immense peace and happiness," continued the old lady.

"During his wife's pregnancy, he came across the ancient scriptures of Garbh Sanskar. That inspired him deeply. He realized that this miraculous knowledge is getting lost with time. So, he took up the cause of sharing it with the world because he firmly believes that Garbh Sanskar is one of the ways to make this world a better place to live."

"He takes these sessions for free because he doesn't want any mother to be deprived of this knowledge due to economic constraints."

Ananya's eyes were filled with respect.

"He is a simple man whose purpose in life is to work towards the betterment of society. He conducts these sessions thrice a year and he has trained more than ten lakh women across the world till now. At other times, he acts as a trustee for various trusts and spends time in NGOs working to provide education to poor children and protecting the environment."

The old lady paused and drank water. "He is a wonderful man, born to serve the world. He has found his higher purpose and he inspires others to find their purpose in life."

Ananya had newfound admiration for the Ancient Guru. *It's not easy to dedicate one's life to a higher purpose.* Ananya was proud of her Guru. Also, now she knew who was the owner of the super-luxury car. She would have never guessed it. She felt blessed to have him in her life. She was determined to follow his teachings and become the best version of herself.

She thanked the old lady and left.

DO IT RIGHT

1. A baby craves attention and love.
2. Garbh Samvad means talking to your baby. When you talk to your baby, he feels loved and valued. He will develop a healthy emotional quotient and will be full of love.
3. Our words have power. They transmit energy. Be very careful about what you share through your words. Don't talk about negative things with your baby.
4. One can only share what they have in abundance and not when they lack it. Fill yourself with love to give love to your baby.
5. Nurture a deeper bond with your baby through Garbh Samvad.
6. Our body has thousands of energy points, but 107 points are major energy points. By stimulating these energy points gently, all the blockages and toxins accumulated in that region are removed and prana begins to flow freely again. It is called Marma therapy.
7. Examples of marma are – blessing someone, peacock feathers treatment, wrestling warm-up, self-defense, greeting namaste, etc.
8. Become your best version and give birth to a baby who can impact the whole world and work towards the betterment of society
9. Garbh Sanskar is not easy but it's the right thing to do.

CHAPTER 10
THE CHALLENGE

Ananya and Riya were determined to become their best versions and implement everything taught by the Ancient Guru. They met daily and continued their daily rituals without fail. They often mentioned the Ancient Guru and how badly they missed the sessions, but it didn't weaken them. The strong memories of Ancient Guru filled them with energy and strengthen their commitment. The sisterhood bond between them grew stronger with each passing day. They even started talking to each other's babies and introduced them in their baby album as sisters. They both have become vital pillars of support for each other. Now they visited the same gynecologist Dr. Rita and had couples meet every weekend to have fun. Their expected date of delivery (EDD) was just a week away from each other.

Ananya shared her library with Riya and made sure she read one book every week. On the other hand, Riya taught Ananya to play the sitar, and she loved it. Ananya was scared earlier and thought she wouldn't be able to learn. But, Riya made it very simple for her and Ananya learned to play in just fifteen days.

Ananya wrote a book titled '*Courtroom Experiences*' and it was widely appreciated in the legal field. It was a collection of experiences from different cases along with key learnings. It aimed to help all the new law students in their practice.

Riya wrote a collection of short stories with morals for kids. It became Amazon's bestseller within a month. The author's community of the city awarded her the best storyteller of the year. She felt blessed to have Ananya by her side, who motivated her to complete her book and conveyed her gratitude to keep her motivated. Ananya complimented her back for her hard work and her connection with babies.

Ananya's terrace was now filled with over thirty plants. She loved her terrace more after the makeover. It had various plants ranging from money plant, tulsi, mint, peppermint, red rose, hibiscus, aloe vera, neem, arbi, tomato, turmeric, green chilies, morning glory, etc. She loved the red rose the most. Whenever it matured, she cut it gently and present it to Arjun in the morning with a gentle kiss and a red rose. She had even hung a cardboard nest for the sparrow to lay eggs. The sparrow hasn't made it its home yet, but Riya and Ananya kept hoping for it and were optimistic that it would.

Five months later

Ananya's baby kicked first at the beginning of the 5th month. In contrast, Riya's baby started kicking at the beginning of the 6th month.

Now, Riya and Ananya were in the 7th month of their pregnancy. After their morning rituals, Riya declared, "Ananya, it's the 7th month now."

"Yes! Is there anything special?" said Ananya, trying to put up a serious face.

"As if you don't know Ananya. Stop being so naïve Ananya," Riya chuckled.

Ananya knew very well that Riya was talking about the photoshoot. She just loved teasing Riya.

Ananya kept giving an 'I don't know' look and Riya shrugged her shoulders.

"Okay, relax. I know you are talking about the photoshoot," acknowledged Ananya.

Riya's eyes widened with a puppy smile on her face. "Yes!" she exclaimed.

"Let's have it this weekend?" Ananya suggested.

Riya agreed instantly and they started discussing the dresses. They wanted to do their maternity photoshoot in that same park – Greenland, where they met each other and the Ancient Guru for the first time. Both of them wanted to have nature's effect in their photographs and the place gave them nostalgia. Arjun and Varun joined them for a few couple shots.

Riya and Ananya even posed for sisterhood wearing a floral tiara and making victory symbols.

Ananya also planned a swimming pool shoot, but Riya did not join her as she didn't know how to swim and was scared of water. Ananya did not insist much as it was the 7th month of pregnancy and too much adventure wasn't advisable.

Ananya wore a green mermaid dress for the swimming pool. Arjun also joined her for a few shots. Riya and Varun were chilling on the pool chair and enthusiastically suggesting new poses to Ananya.

The couples spent their fun-filled photoshoot weekend happily and bid each other goodbye.

Two months later

Ananya and Riya started their 9th month practice of affirmations and **Apana mudra** for normal delivery. Riya was finding it difficult to exercise, but Ananya kept encouraging her. They enjoyed partner workouts the most. They did yoga, 100 squats, pranayamas and meditations daily.

At the beginning of Ananya's 9th month, they went to Dr. Rita's clinic for a routine checkup. Ananya's sonography reports were a little complicated. The amniotic fluid index (AFI) was very low. Dr. Rita prescribed her the medications and asked her to keep a tap on the baby's movements. Ananya shared this with Arjun. Arjun consoled her and assured her that everything would be fine. Riya also reassured Ananya and advised her not to stress. They both went to the temple to pray for their babies and smooth delivery process.

Ananya started to research about the low AFI and tried various acupressure points to increase the fluid. After a week, Ananya and Arjun went to Dr. Rita's clinic. The AFI was still low. The doctor suggested that they will wait for another week and do sonography again. A caesarean will be the only option if the condition doesn't change. The couple was upset. The couple took the opinion of two other gynecologists and both concurred on the caesarean decision. Ananya wanted a normal delivery. Arjun said it was okay. All we want is healthy delivery of the baby with utmost safety. The method doesn't matter much.

"Can we ask the Ancient Guru about this?" Ananya suggested.

Arjun was reluctant at first but couldn't refuse Ananya. They went to the Ancient Guru's office the same day. And surprisingly, he was in Mumbai at that time for a business meeting. Ananya and Arjun were waiting at the reception. Ananya was very excited to meet the Ancient Guru personally. Soon they were called into his meeting room.

The Ancient Guru wore a formal shirt and trousers. Ananya felt an instant lift in her energy in his presence. She knew she was at the right place.

The Ancient Guru greeted the couple and listened to their problem attentively. He suggested marma therapy for the next three days.

"The marma points which I had taught were just the tip of the iceberg. Several other points have tremendous health benefits. Generally, pregnant women face low hemoglobin issues. We have seen that the hemoglobin levels rise by one point instantly just after the marma therapy. Even in cases of low AFI, the fluid is restored in most cases within a few sessions. But for the treatment to work, you need to have complete faith in it and no stress is allowed. We can try our best and hold faith in the higher energies to work in our favor," said the Ancient Guru.

Ananya nodded and decided to take the marma sessions on that day itself. Ananya and Arjun thanked the Ancient Guru and went to the Marma Chikitsha clinic recommended by him.

"Do you want to take marma sessions?" asked Arjun. *I am not sure if it will be helpful.*

"Yes, I trust him completely. And there is no harm in trying whatever is possible," replied Ananya.

They reached the Marma Chikitsha clinic and Ananya was called into the therapy room. She was a little nervous and wanted things to get normal soon. She hated this anxiety. She instantly found the atmosphere of the room to be peaceful. She loved the soothing fragrance of the room and the ignited oil lamp worked as a source of strength and hope for her.

After a few moments, the old lady entered the therapy room. She was the same lady who had told her about the Ancient Guru. Ananya started crying in front of her. The lady passed a tissue box and asked her to relax.

185

"Marma Therapy heals our subtle body. By stimulating the marma points, we remove the toxins that have accumulated in our gross body and enable the free flow of prana. When the prana flows freely, our gross body heals itself and becomes healthy again. This marma therapy has helped in increasing hemoglobin, regulating AFI, relieving stress and promoting overall well-being in pregnant women," explained the old lady.

The old lady asked Ananya to lie on the bed and close her eyes. She placed her hands on her head and began giving the marma therapy by chanting a few mantras. Ananya loved the soothing sound of the chants and tried to surrender all her stresses to the divine. The old lady sensed the tension in her body and whispered to not get stressed and relax completely. Ananya couldn't drop her focus altogether. After all, thinking about a caesarean scared the hell out of her. She wanted the best for her baby. Even marma therapy couldn't relax her restless mind completely. It gave her relief, but the relief was short-lived. Because of stress, Ananya could not have that experience she had on the stage. But it was helpful and she felt calmer.

The subsequent sessions in the following days relaxed her even more. In her fourth session, she could feel the baby moving very fast and had an out of world experience. She was finally able to relax after a stressful week. The tension on her face was eased to a great extent. The glow was back on her face.

After a week the couple went to Dr. Rita's clinic for sonography to take the final decision.

Ananya was lying on the bed for sonography with her fingers crossed. Dr. Rita followed the procedure and double-checked the screen. She was taken aback. *This must be the work of the Ancient Guru.*

She told the couple that the AFI was back to normal now, which is no less than a miracle. Both mother and baby are healthy now. We can wait for labor pain to be induced naturally.

"Ananya, tell me your secret? How did you do it?" Dr. Rita asked.

Ananya told her about the Ancient Guru's guidance and Marma therapy. Dr. Rita had heard about his energy healing methods, but she got to experience it herself today. Healing through faith and energy alignment is a rarity these days. Indeed, the power of the subconscious mind is unlimited.

"He is truly the blessed one and is doing commendable work guiding young mothers," said Dr. Rita.

Dr. Rita congratulated the couple and wished them all the best.

After a week, Ananya finally noticed a sparrow making a nest in the cardboard house. She was delighted. Her wait had lasted over eight months and now a sparrow was finally there on her terrace. She was content. Eventually, everything was falling back into place – her AFI and now the sparrow too. She called Arjun to show him the sparrow and hugged him tightly.

Just as she was feeling snug, she felt a sharp pain in her pelvis. Stress lines replaced the pleasure on her face.

Arjun felt Ananya tensed up. He asked, "What's wrong?"

"I don't know. I am suddenly feeling pain in my pelvis," lamented Ananya.

"Come, take a seat," guided Arjun.

Arjun called Dr. Rita and she suggested that it can be labor pain and asked them to note down the *duration and frequency* of the pain.

"When the pain is very intense and frequent, you must come to the hospital," explained Dr. Rita.

Arjun thanked the doctor and explained it to Ananya. She was happy that the day had come when she could finally hold her baby in her arms.

She called Riya and told her about the labor pain. Riya and Varun soon came to her house to encourage and divert her attention. *Dr. Rita had suggested that they do light dance and listen to soothing music during labor to ease the pain*, Riya recalled. She enthusiastically turned on the music and pulled Ananya's hand. Ananya stood up and they danced gently. Arjun and Varun also joined them. Ananya loved Riya's idea and she was able to dance through the pain.

Their bodies were tired but their souls were revitalized. Ananya's pain became sharper and more frequent. With contractions coming in less than 5-minute intervals and she knew she had to now rush to the hospital. All four of them reached the hospital at 6 a.m. and Ananya was taken to the labor room. Dr. Rita was already in the labor room. She supported Ananya and was helping her deliver the baby.

Arjun was breathlessly pacing across the corridor of the hospital. He was filled with anxiety and was murmuring prayers. Varun stopped him, put his hand on Arjun's shoulder and told him not to stress out and that everything will be fine.

Suddenly, the labor room was echoing the cries of the newborn.

"It's a baby boy!" Dr. Rita announced and congratulated Ananya.

The nurse gave the baby to Arjun after cleaning and wrapping him in a blue cloth. Arjun had tears of joy flowing when he held his baby for the first time.

Arjun kissed the baby's forehead gently and whispered, "Welcome to this world, my love!"

Riya and Varun congratulated them. Ananya was shifted to the patient's room to take rest.

As soon as she settled in her room, she asked the nurse and Arjun to put the baby on her chest for breast crawl. The baby had a round face, soft hair and sharp nails. He weighed 3.2 kilograms. Ananya requested Riya to be by her side. Ananya guided the baby to reach the nipple. The baby was moving his hands and legs, trying to adjust to the new atmosphere. He looked adorable and enchanting. His eyes were still half-closed. Within a few minutes, using his stepping reflex, the baby was able to successfully lick the nipple with his mouth. Arjun and Riya were delighted and they clapped lightly.

Then the nurse gently lifted the baby and put him in the cot beside Ananya. Arjun called Varun inside the room. Varun saw the baby and gave him a flying kiss. *Babies are so adorable and full of innocence,* he thought.

Riya was sitting near Ananya and was talking with the newborn baby. Ananya asked her, "when are you bringing your baby to this world?"

"You can ask the baby yourself," Riya answered, pointing towards her womb.

Ananya placed her hand on Riya's womb and whispered, "Come into this beautiful world whenever you feel ready."

Riya suddenly started to feel the sensations in her pelvis and realized that her water broke.

Varun immediately called the doctor and Riya was taken to the doctor's cabin by the nurse. When Dr. Rita checked Riya, she found that Riya had dilated ten centimeters already. *It's surprising how some women don't feel labor pain,* Dr. Rita thought. She was rushed to the labor room. Riya could recall the important teaching of the Ancient Guru that the newborn should be given to the mother immediately after delivery even before cleaning, to press against her warm chest. The baby feels safe and warm in skin-to-skin contact with his mother. She requested Dr. Rita to give her baby immediately for breast crawl and Dr. Rita agreed. Dr. Rita told the nurse that they didn't have time to give an enema. She asked Riya to sit in a squatting position and push while taking deep breaths. Riya obeyed her and with the fourth push, the baby was out. She delivered a baby boy as well. The breast crawl of Riya's baby was also successful. Several studies suggest that holding the baby immediately after birth can ease the delivery pain, release oxytocin hormones giving the mother and baby a sense of calmness and develops a deeper bond between the mother and baby[lvii].

Ananya and Arjun could hear the cries of the newborn. They congratulated Varun and Riya.

Arjun and Varun opted for a bigger room as both the mothers wanted to stay together. Riya's baby had chubby cheeks and curly hair. He weighed 2.8 kilograms and had rashes on his nose, making it look pink in color. Varun had brought them some delicious healthy khichdi. After eating their heart's fill, the new moms felt revitalized.

Watching their babies and wives, the husbands felt delighted. They embraced and congratulated each other. They expressed gratitude to the divine for healthy babies.

Arjun and Varun asked the new moms to hold the babies in their arms and sit close to each other for photos. They even laid the babies on the bed and made a short video. All four of them enjoyed clicking pictures and were cherishing one of the biggest events of their lives.

It had been four hours since Riya's delivery. Both Ananya and Riya were well rested by now and were ready to be discharged.

Riya said excitedly to Ananya, "Wow! our babies are born on the same day."

"Yes, it's the divines' blessing," Ananya said cheerfully. "Happy motherhood, Riya!!"

"Yes! Happy motherhood to a new mom in you, Ananya," congratulated Riya. "He is so connected to you."

Ananya smiled and looked at both the babies. Her baby was looking at everything around him and Riya's baby was sleeping. She looked deep into his eyes and said, "You are just like I imagined you to be. Thank you so much for coming into our lives. How lucky are you! You have a twin best friend already."

"We will continue to strive to be our best versions for them," promised Ananya.

"Yes! Ananya. I promise too. We shall continue with our rituals and read books on parenting for their best growth," said Riya with determination.

"This makes us a perfect family," asserted Ananya.

All of them hugged each other tightly.

Soon, both of them were discharged and they left for home to begin their new journey of parenthood.

JUHI SOHAL

EPILOGUE

Ananya's son had just become one of the youngest renowned **Grandmaster (GM)** by winning World Rapid Chess Championship conducted under the International Chess Federation FIDE. He made his parents and his country proud through his genius. Ananya and Arjun's joy knew no bounds. Deep inside, Ananya was taken back to her pregnancy journey. She mentally thanked Dr. Rita and the Ancient Guru. She was filled with gratitude for her decision to learn and practice Garbh Sanskar. She felt like all her efforts had paid off as she gave her best efforts during her pregnancy and her son Jay had been such a wonderful child. He received the gold medal on the stage in Exhibition Centre, Dubai. Ananya and Arjun clicked his pictures as they cheered him from the crowd.

Riya and Varun watched it live at their home on the news channel. They were very happy with Jay's achievement. Riya called Ananya, congratulated her on Jay's victory, and made all the arrangements for their grand welcome. The décor, the food, the dress, everything was decided. After all, they were like extended family now.

Krishiv, son of Riya and Varun, won various singing competitions at the school, city, district, and state levels. He has been a very successful YouTuber as well. He had recently crossed the one million subscribers landmark on his channel just at the age of seven years through his singing videos.

Krishiv's singing was everyone's favorite at all the events and parties. Everyone loved to listen to his pure and soothing voice. Maybe it was the magic of Riya's sitar or may the blessings of Ancient Guru, they always wondered. Riya would often accompany him by playing sitar while he sang.

Krishiv was very delighted on learning about Jay's victory. For Jay's grand victory, he wanted to write a song, dedicating it to him. He asked for help from his ever-supportive parents and they agreed. Soon, they came up with a song and were all set to welcome Jay, Ananya and Arjun.

Appendix 1
GARBH SANSKAR RITUALS

RITUAL #1: Pray to Divine Daily

RITUAL #2: Create Your Baby Album And Read It Daily

RITUAL #3: Know Your Most Authentic Self

RITUAL #4: Eat Consciously Every Time

RITUAL #5: Heal Your Chakras

RITUAL #6: Practice Nine Rounds Of Anulom Vilom Pranayama Daily

RITUAL #7: Practice Mudra Pranayama Daily

RITUAL #8: Spend Time With Nature Daily

RITUAL #9: Listen To Music Every Day

RITUAL #10: Engage Yourself In Creativity

RITUAL #11: Solve Puzzles Daily

RITUAL #12: Feed Your Soul By Reading Books Daily

RITUAL #13: Talk To Your Baby Daily

RITUAL #14: Give Yourself Marma Daily (Pg)76)

Appendix 2
BECOME A SUPERMOM!

The end of this book is the beginning of your journey towards becoming a supermom.

Garbh Sanskar is an ancient technique that changes lives and has the potential to change the whole generation. One mother can impact the world in so many ways. Every mother is just one decision away to be the source of change to make this world a better place to live.

Garbh Sanskar isn't just a set of few activities. Garbh Sanskar is every thought you think, every emotion you feel, every action you take, every habit you create, every energy you generate and every food you eat. It's a lifestyle. It's a mindset. **Garbh Sanskar is not easy, but it's the right thing to do.**

When Garbh Sanskar is inculcated under proper guidance, the world benefits from such determined mothers. Those mothers can create history through their divine womb.

You are here because you are chosen by the divine. All the best for your motherhood journey!

I would love to hear from you at officialsupermoms@gmail.com

ABOUT THE AUTHOR

Juhi Sohal is a Garbh Sanskar coach and a certified yoga practitioner trained at the Sri Sri School of Yoga. She is a free-spirited person who believes in alternative healing sciences.

She is a mother of a one-year-old baby boy and loves to read and learn new things. She is a yogi, a marma practitioner, a productivity coach, a gardener, a nature lover and a fitness enthusiast.

She founded Supermoms – let's create a better world in 2021 to help one million couples experience the miracles of Garbh Sanskar and make this world a better place.

Today, we live in an aggressive, mentally disturbed, and violent world. Juhi believes that the most effective way to change the world is to sow the right seeds during conception and pregnancy. By following Garbh Sanskar, a mother can give birth to a genius baby, full of virtues, balanced from within, happy, satisfied, a peace lover, and who works towards the betterment of the world at large.

Garbh Sanskar can be followed by planning and expecting mothers for the baby's best development. It's their journey from ordinary to extraordinary, to give their all in attracting a genius baby and serving humankind through their motherhood.

REFERENCES

[i] Sandra Ackerman. *Discovering the Brain*. Chapter 6.

[ii] Dr. G. Vijayalakshmi (August. 2017). *Mother - The Architect of Child*. IOSR-JHSS. Volume 22. Issue 8. Ver. I. pp 73-78.

Jyotsna Deshpande. (2013). *The Effect of Selected Aspect of Garbha Sanskar on Stress, Coping Strategies and Wellbeing of Antenatal Mothers*. IJSR.

[iii] Jyotsna Singh. (2018). *Garbhsanskar Mental and Intellectual Development of Unborn Child*. Journal of Neonatal Studies. Vol 1. Issue 1.

Priyanka Hajare, Bharathi K, Pushpalatha B and Hetal Dave. (2019). *Garbha Sanskar- Need of Every Expectant Mother For Healthy Progeny*. Int J Recent Sci Res. 10(11), pp. 36140-36143.

[iv] *Garbha Upanishad*, Krishna Yajur Veda

[v] Centre on the Developing Child. Harvard university. *Genetics and child development*. DOI: https://developingchild.harvard.edu/resources/what-is-epigenetics-and-how-does-it-relate-to-child-development/

[vi] Suresh Alka Prajapati. (2018). *Garbhsanskar*. ISBN: 978-93-82345-98-5

[vii] Prof K.R. Srikantha Murthy. *Astanga Hrdayam*

[viii] Imagine the universe. *Superstrings*. National Aeronautics and Space Administration. DOI: https://imagine.gsfc.nasa.gov/science/questions/superstring.html

Christopher S. Reynolds, M. C. David Marsh, Helen R. Russell, Andrew C. Fabian, Robyn Smith, Francesco Tombesi and Sylvain Veilleux. (2022 February 12). *Astrophysical Limits on Very Light Axion-like Particles from Chandra Grating Spectroscopy of NGC 1275*. The Astrophysical Journal. DOI: https://iopscience.iop.org/article/10.3847/1538-4357/ab6a0c

[ix]Irishtimes. (2011 February 17). *The pseudoscience of creating beautiful (or ugly) water.* DOI: https://www.irishtimes.com/news/science/the-pseudoscience-of-creating-beautiful-or-ugly-water-1.574583

[x] Emoto M. (1999) *Messages from Water,* HADO Kyoikusha Co., Ltd. Tokyo. 2001. ISBN 4-939098-00-1

[xi]Jack Kornfield. *The Art of Forgiveness, Lovingkindness, and Peace*

Melanie Lidman. (2014). *African tradition blends with religion to illuminate path to forgiveness.*

[xii] Rhonda Byrne. (2012). *The Magic.* ISBN: 978-1-84983-839-9

[xiii] Prof. Dr. Jeetendra Adhia. (2008). *Prayer of Mind.* Adhia International.

[xiv] Rhonda Byrne. (2010). *The Power.* ISBN: 978-0-85720-170-6

[xv] Claude M. Briston. (1969). *The Magic of Believing.* ISBN: 978-0-671-74521-9

[xvi] Cain Polidano, Anna Zhu and Joel Bornstein. (2017 Sept 13). *The relation between cesarean birth and child cognitive development.* Sci Rep 7, 11483. DOI: 10.1038/s41598-017-10831-y

Dr. Thomas Verny. (1982). *The secret life of the unborn child.* ISBN: 978-0440505655

[xvii] Rien Verdult. (2009). Caesarean Birth: Psychological Aspects in Babies. Int. J. Prenatal and Perinatal Psychology and Medicine Vol. 21, No. 1/2, pp. 29–49. DOI: http://www.mattes.de/buecher/praenatale_psychologie/PP_PDF/PP_2 1_1-2_Verdult2.pdf

[xviii] Louise L. Hay. (2005). *You can heal your life.* ISBN:978-81-905655-8-5

[xix] Dr. Joseph Murphy. (2012) *The Power of your Subconscious Mind. ISBN: 978-93-80227-58-0.*

[xx] Geeta Press. *Srimad Bhagwad Gita.* Gorakhpur

xxi Sri Sri Paramahansa Yogananda. (2002). *The Bhagavad Gita.* Vol I. pp 281.

xxii Sir Edwin Arnold. (2014). *The Bhagavad Gita,* 4th impression. pp 20.

xxiii Sutrasthanas'. *Charaka Samhita.* Chapter 27.

xxiv Colleen de Bellefonds. (2021 May 14). *When babies develop taste buds and start tasting food.* DOI: https://www.whattoexpect.com/pregnancy/fetal-development/fetal-taste/

Arlene Eisenberg and Heidi Murkoff. *What to Expect When You're Expecting & What to Eat When You're Expecting*

xxv Dr. Shri Balaji Tambe. (2019). *Ayurvedic Garbh Sanskar.* ISBN: 978-93-80571-87-4

xxvi Recommended and verified by *Dr. Chandrakant Amdavadi (B.A.M.S)*, an Ayurvedic Doctor with over 20 years of experience and an expert speaker on Sri Sri Tattva Panel.

xxvii Peter Malakoff. (2005). *Light on Ayurveda.* Journal of Health. DOI: https://www.ancientorganics.com/ghee-a-short-consideration-from-an-ayurvedic-perspective/

xxviii M.S. Anu, Suprabha Kunjibettu, S. Archana and Laxmipriya Dei. (2017). *Management of Premature Contractions through Shatavaryadi Ksheerapaka Basti.* DOI: https://www.ncbi.nlm.nih.gov/pmc/articles/PMC6153909/

xxix Recommended and verified by Botanist *Nimila Kanth (M.Sc.)* with over 15 years of experience

xxx Shree Gulabkunverba Ayurvedic Society. (1949). *Charaka Samhita*

xxxi Recommended and verified by *Dr. Deepa Kaushik (B.A.M.S),* an Ayurvedic Doctor with over 15 years of experience and a Garbh Sanskar Coach

xxxii World Health Organisation. (2019) *Microplastics in drinking water.* ISBN 978-92-4-151619-8. DOI: https://apps.who.int/iris/rest/bitstreams/1243269/retrieve

xxxiii Sri Sri Paramahansa Yogananda. (2002). *The Bhagavad Gita*. Vol I. pp 477 Chapter 4 Verse 24, and Vol II. Pp 947 Chapter 15 Verse 14. DOI: http://saibaba.ws/prayers/brahmaarpanam.htm

xxxiv Dr.Marc Halpern. *Principles of Ayurvedic Medicines.*

Paramahansa Yogananda. (1998). *Autobiography of a Yogi*

xxxv Swami Muktibodhananda (1998) *Hatha Yoga Pradipika*. pp 160

xxxvi Pancham Sinh. *Hatha Yoga Pradipika*

xxxvii B.K.S Iyengar. (2014). *Light on Yoga*. ISBN: 978-81-7223501-7

xxxviii Dilip Sarkar.*Yoga Therapy for Health and Healing of Body Mind and Spirit*

xxxix Swami Muktibodhananda (1998) *Hatha Yoga Pradipika*. pp 283

xl National Library of Medicine. (2019). *Sound perception in plants.*

Osmania University. (2014) *Effect of Different Types of Music on Rosa Chinensis Plants*

xli South Korea's National Institute of Agricultural Biotechnology. (2018). *Beyond chemical triggers.*

xlii Paramahansa Yogananda. (1998). *Autobiography of a Yogi*

xliii Ajay Anil Gurjar, Siddharth Ladkake & Ajay Thakare (2009 January). *Analysis of Acoustic of OM chant to study its effect on nervous system*. IJCSNS Vol 9 No.1. DOI: http://paper.ijcsns.org/07_book/200901/20090151.pdf

xliv Ravindra Arya, Maya Chandsoria, Ramesh Konanki, Dillep Tiwari. (2012 February 14). *Maternal Music Exposure during Pregnancy Influences Neonatal Behaviour: An Open-Label Randomized Controlled Trial*. DOI: https://www.hindawi.com/journals/ijpedi/2012/901812/

xlv Satavisa Pati. (2021 September 1). *Adoption of sanskrit by NASA aims to change the language of GAP*. DOI:

https://www.analyticsinsight.net/adoption-of-sanskrit-by-nasa-aims-to-change-the-language-gap/

xlvi Elena Racevska and Meri Tadlnac. (2018 May). *Intelligence, music preferences, and uses of music from the perspective of evolutionary psychology.* Evolutionary Behavioral Sciences. DOI: https://doi.apa.org/doiLanding?doi=10.1037%2Febs0000124

xlvii Rauscher, Frances and others. (1994). *Music and spatial task performance: a causal relationship.* Journal Nature.

xlviii David Code. (2010). *To Raise Happy Kids, Put Your Marriage First.*

xlix Denise Mann. (2013 January 3). *Babies listen and learn while in the womb.* DOI: https://www.webmd.com/baby/news/20130102/babies-learn-womb#1

Acta Paediatrica. (2012). *Newborn memories of the "oohs" and "ahs" heard in the womb*

l Recommended and verified by *Dr. Deepa Kaushik (B.A.M.S),* an Ayurvedic Doctor with over 15 years of experience and a Garbh Sanskar Coach

li Emoto, Masaru. (2004). *The Hidden Messages in Water.* Atria Books. pp 90-91

Karen Carnabucci. (2018). *3 jars of rice.* DOI: https://www.realtruekaren.com/blog/3-jars-of-rice-plus-love-and-hate-equals-an-amazing-experiment

lii Murthy KRS. *Susruta Samhita.*Volume I, II, III.

National Health Portal. (2015 September 28). *Marma Therapy.* DOI: https://www.nhp.gov.in/marma-therapy_mtl

liii Joshi SK. *Marma Science and Principles of Marma Therapy*

livDr.Vasant Lad and Anisha Durve. (2016 Jan 1). *Marma Points of Ayurveda.* ISBN: 978-1883725198

Pooja Sabharwal, Vartika kashyap, Gaur, M.B., Yogesh Pandey and Gaurav Phull. (2018). "Physio-pathological study of Migraine & its Pacification with Marma Chikitsa", International Journal of Development Research, 8, (06), 21193-21198.   DOI: https://www.journalijdr.com/sites/default/files/issue-pdf/13419.pdf

Dr.S.H.Acharya. (2014 Jan 1). *Science of Marma*. ISBN: 978-0980002928

[lv] Recommended and verified by *Dr. Hemant Sharma (B.A.M.S)*, an Ayurvedic Doctor with over 20 years of experience and a Marma Therapy Coach

[lvi] Dr. Avinash Lele, Dr Subhash Ranade and Dr. David Frawley. (2009 Dec 31). Secret*s of Marma: The Lost Secrets of Ayurveda*. ISBN: 978-8170841777

[lvii] UNICEF, WHO. *Capture the Moment – Early initiation of breastfeeding: The best start for every newborn.* New York: UNICEF; 2018. DOI: https://www.unicef.org/eca/media/4256/file/Capture-the-moment-EIBF-report.pdf

Dr.Varsha Tiwari, Dr.Neelam Singh, Dr. Ashish Purohit and Dr. Saroj Shyam. (2015 June 16). *Role of breast crawl in maternal health and well-being.* Int J Med Res Rev 2015;3(6):540-546. DOI: https://ijmrr.medresearch.in/index.php/ijmrr/article/view/277/540

Made in the USA
Las Vegas, NV
09 November 2023

80515604R00132